W9-AWZ-001

American Heart Association®

Fighting Heart Disease and Stroke

Heartsaver CPR

A COMPREHENSIVE COURSE FOR THE LAY RESPONDER

Adult, Infant, and Child

Cardiopulmonary Resuscitation

and First Aid for Choking

ISBN 0-87493-317-X

If you want to know what to do in an emergency, the American Heart Association (AHA) Heartsaver CPR courses can help you. With the knowledge and skills you learn in these courses, you can save the life of a loved one, a friend, a coworker, or a citizen in your community.

These new courses are for the lay rescuer who needs a credential (a card) documenting successful completion of a CPR course. Such credentials are often required in the workplace. This course will prepare you to respond to emergencies in the workplace as part of an emergency response system. You can then serve as a lay responder.

These courses will teach you how to recognize and treat life-threatening emergencies, including cardiac arrest and choking. You also will learn to recognize the warning signs of heart attack and stroke in adults and signs of breathing difficulty in children. By recognizing these signs and phoning 911 (or other emergency response number in your area), you may save a life.

This manual may be used to teach any 1 of 3 Heartsaver CPR courses for lay rescuers:

Course 1: Adult CPR teaches warning signs of heart attack and stroke, CPR, and relief of choking for adult victims. Course 1 uses only Module 1.

Course 2: Infant and Child CPR teaches prevention of injuries and cardiac arrest, CPR, and relief of choking for infants (birth to 1 year of age) and children (1 to 8 years of age). Course 2 uses only Module 2.

Course 3: CPR for All Ages teaches CPR and relief of choking for adult, infant, and child victims. This course uses both Module 1 and Module 2.

This manual is divided into 2 modules:

Module 1: Adult CPR — Page 1	Module 2: Infant and Child CPR — Page 67
Module 1 includes information about warning signs of heart attack and stroke, CPR, and relief of choking (foreign-body airway obstruction) for adult and child victims 8 years of age and older.	**Module 2** includes information about prevention of injuries and cardiac arrest, CPR, and relief of choking (foreign-body airway obstruction) for infant and child victims up to 8 years of age.

This student manual contains several features designed to help you learn CPR, including *learning objectives, review questions,* and *skills review* sheets. These components will help make learning easier. At the start of each chapter, read the learning objectives carefully. This will help you focus on the essential information in each chapter. When you finish reading the chapter, answer the review questions. If you cannot answer a question or if you choose the wrong answer, review the parts of the chapter related to that question.

This manual also contains colored boxes that highlight important and useful information. The red boxes contain Critical Concepts, information that is *essential* for mastering the knowledge and skills taught in this course. Critical signs and symptoms included in these red boxes or elsewhere in the text are called red flags. The blue boxes contain Foundation Facts, which explain or justify actions and recommendations and provide important supportive information. The black boxes are FYI..., information that may be of interest to some course participants but is *not* required to fulfill the core learning objectives.

The skills performance sheets ("Performance Criteria") in the appendixes of Modules 1 and 2 list the skills you will practice in class. To obtain a *Course Completion Card* at the end of this course, you must complete a written examination satisfactorily and demonstrate each skill listed on the skills performance sheet to your instructor. Review each skill, pay attention to the details, and practice carefully. This manual will be a valuable resource for you before, during, and after your training. It is easy to forget some CPR skills, so practice the skills and reread this manual after you complete the course.

The appendixes also contain case scenarios to help you apply your knowledge of CPR to real-life situations. The appendixes include answers to frequently asked questions about CPR, special situations in CPR, self-test questions, and a glossary of terms. This information is provided to help you learn faster and integrate your knowledge after reading the manual. Take advantage of this information to prepare yourself for the course and acquire the skills to save a life.

For more information about interventions to reduce the risk of injury and updated recommendations on the steps of CPR, visit the AHA website at *www.americanheart.org*. This site contains links to other sites with useful information.

We wish you success as you learn CPR. When you complete the course, you will be better prepared to recognize the warning signs of emergencies in adults, to prevent many causes of cardiac arrest in infants and children, and to respond to future emergencies by using the skills of CPR.

Module 1 Adult CPR

Chapter **1** *Early Action Saves Lives*
The Chain of Survival and Warning Signs of Heart Attack and Stroke

Chapter **1** *Early Action Saves Lives*

*The Chain of Survival and Warning
Signs of Heart Attack and Stroke*

Case Scenario, Option 1

*You are walking on a beach, and you see a
family enjoying a picnic near the water. An
elderly man, a middle-aged man, and 2 children
are sitting on a blanket eating lunch. As you
walk by, you overhear some of the conversation,
allowing you to identify a grandfather, a father,
a 3-year-old son, and a 10-month-old son. You
speak briefly to them and then continue walking.
Suddenly you hear someone shout from the
direction you have come, "Help! I think he needs
CPR! I don't know what to do! Somebody help
me!" As you run toward the shout, you realize
it came from the area of the family picnic. You
wonder who needs CPR. Is it the grandfather,
the father, the 3-year-old child, or the infant?*

Who in the family is the most likely victim of
cardiopulmonary arrest? What actions should
you be prepared to take for that victim?

By the end of this module you will be able to
identify the most likely causes of sudden cardiac
arrest in adults and how to recognize the signs
of heart attack and stroke.

Case Scenario, Option 1, continued

*You run to the scene of the picnic. The family
is gathered around the father, who is clearly in
distress. He is pale and sweaty and complains of
nausea. He says he has terrible chest discomfort
that he describes as a tightness or pressure.
He says that the chest discomfort feels like it
is moving to his neck, jaw, and left arm. He
tells you that the discomfort has lasted for*

*10 minutes. You offer to call an ambulance, but
he says, "No, I think it's just indigestion from the
barbecue," and he asks you to get him an
antacid tablet.*

What problem is this man likely to be experiencing?
Why is it important to take action? What action
should you take?

Case Scenario, Option 2

*You return to the scene of the picnic. The family
is gathered around the grandfather. He looks ill,
and one side of his face droops as he tries to
speak. His right arm hangs uselessly by his side,
and he is unable to walk. You ask him if he is
OK, and he replies with very slurred words that
his head hurts and "something's wrong."*

What problem is this man likely to be experiencing?
Why is it important to take action? What action
should you take?

Learning Objectives

After reading this chapter you should be able to

1. Name the links in the AHA adult Chain of
   Survival and discuss the role *you* play in the
   Chain of Survival.

2. List the warning signs of these 4 major adult
   emergencies:

   a. Heart attack
   b. Cardiac arrest
   c. Stroke
   d. Choking (foreign-body airway obstruction)
      in the responsive adult

Cardiovascular Disease and How YOU Can Help

Cardiovascular disease is the single greatest cause of death in the United States. Every year more than 480,000 adult Americans die of a **heart attack** or related complications. About half of these deaths (some 225,000) result from **sudden cardiac arrest**. Sudden cardiac arrest can complicate a heart attack. If it does, it is most likely to occur during the *first hour* after the onset of symptoms of a heart attack, typically before the victim arrives at the hospital. Sudden cardiac arrest will result in death unless emergency treatment is provided immediately.

The victim of an emergency such as a heart attack, cardiac arrest, stroke, or choking may be saved if people at the scene start the **Chain of Survival**. In this chapter you will learn the critical actions that make up the 4 links in the AHA adult Chain of Survival. You will learn how to recognize the symptoms of these 4 emergencies. You will learn when to phone 911 (or other emergency response number in your area), when and how to perform CPR, and when and how to attempt to relieve choking in adults.

AHA Chain of Survival

The AHA Chain of Survival symbol **(see Figure 1)** depicts the critical actions required to treat life-threatening emergencies, including heart attack, cardiac arrest, stroke, and choking.

Once you recognize an emergency, you should *immediately*

- **Phone 911** (or other emergency response number) to activate the emergency medical services (EMS) system
- **Begin CPR**

The next 2 links will be provided by rescuers with additional training:

- **Early defibrillation** by trained rescuers or EMS personnel
- **Advanced care** by EMS and hospital personnel

You must know when to activate the Chain of Survival. You must recognize when an emergency exists. When you recognize the emergency, the first 2 links—**phone 911** (or other emergency response number) and **begin CPR**—are in your hands. *You* perform the actions or links that increase a victim's chance of survival. Skilled rescuers and emergency professionals will respond to the 911 emergency call. They will be trained and equipped to provide defibrillation and advanced care to further increase the victim's chance of survival.

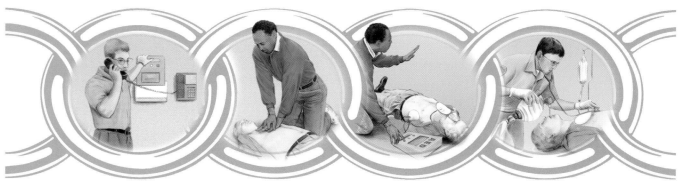

© 1998 American Heart Association

FIGURE 1. *The AHA Adult Chain of Survival.* The 4 links or sets of actions in the chain are **(1)** phone 911, **(2)** CPR, **(3)** early defibrillation, and **(4)** advanced care.

To save people with heart attack, cardiac arrest, or stroke, *each set of actions or link in the Chain of Survival must be performed as soon as possible*. If any link in the chain is weak, delayed, or missing, the chance of survival is lessened. The 4 links in the Chain of Survival are discussed below.

First Link: Phone 911

The first set of actions in the treatment of any emergency is recognizing that an emergency exists and phoning 911 or other emergency response number in your area. You must recognize the warning signs of a heart attack, cardiac arrest, stroke, or choking. *Anyone* who is *unresponsive* should receive emergency care. Heart attack, cardiac arrest, stroke, and choking can cause the victim to become unresponsive. Although many conditions, not just cardiac arrest, can cause the victim to have no response, *all* victims who suddenly become unresponsive will benefit from activation of the Chain of Survival.

Lay responders often serve as part of an emergency response system in the workplace. If the emergency response system includes an emergency number other than 911, use that number as instructed. The operator who answers this emergency response number should determine your location and the nature of the emergency, phone the local EMS system, and send other trained rescuers who are on-site to help you until EMS personnel arrive. If you are part of a workplace emergency response team, whenever this manual indicates that you should phone 911, you should phone the emergency response number at your workplace.

If your workplace participates in a public access defibrillation (PAD) program, trained rescuers will be on-site to perform CPR and provide early defibrillation with an automated external defibrillator (AED). If your workplace is in a PAD program, when you or another rescuer phones

---

FYI...

Emergency Medical Dispatch Assistance and Enhanced 911

In many areas of the United States emergency medical dispatchers (EMDs) are taught how to help callers give emergency care. The instructions are simple, and they will help you help the victim until EMS personnel arrive.

The EMD can coach you through the basic steps of CPR. If you can bring the phone to the victim's side, follow the EMD's instructions. If other rescuers are at the scene and the EMD provides instructions, stay on the phone and do the following:

- Repeat the dispatcher's instructions loudly to the other rescuers and confirm that they are following each step.
- If the victim vomits or other complications occur, tell the dispatcher. Rescuers are not expected to perform perfectly in such a crisis.
- Be sure that rescuers follow each instruction, even if it takes extra seconds.
- Ensure the safety of the rescuers at all times.
- When EMS personnel arrive at the victim's side, the dispatcher will hang up after confirming their arrival.
- You hang up last or if instructed to do so by the dispatcher.

Find out if your community has *enhanced* 911. In enhanced 911 systems a computer automatically confirms the caller's address. This allows the dispatcher to locate the caller even if the caller is unable to speak or the connection is broken. If your community does not have an enhanced 911 system, you should become a vocal advocate for such services. Enhanced 911 can save precious seconds, minutes, and lives.

the emergency response number, get the AED (usually located near the phone). Place the AED at the victim's side so that it will be available when other trained rescuers arrive.

Other rescuers are often nearby. If you find a person who is unresponsive, shout for help to bring other rescuers to help you. When you or another rescuer calls 911 (or other emergency response number), the dispatcher will ask questions and relay the information you provide to the response team. You should reply with short, specific answers, giving only the requested information. The dispatcher will probably ask:

- **"What is your emergency?"** You might answer: *"My husband had sudden chest pain and has now collapsed."*

- **"What's happening now?"** *"My friend is giving CPR."*

- **"Where is the victim located?"** *"We're at the Evergreen Apartments, 1234 Fifth Avenue Northeast, on the second floor in the back of the building."*

- **"What number are you calling from?"** *"555-1313."* At this point the dispatcher may give you directions such as **"Stay on the line until I tell you to hang up. Rescuers are being sent to your location. Please send someone to meet them and direct them to the scene."**

Second Link: CPR

CPR is a set of actions that the rescuer performs in sequence to *assess and support* airway, breathing, and circulation if needed. CPR is performed in steps **(see Figure 2)** so that the rescuer provides only the support the victim needs.

CPR is the critical link that buys time between the first link (phone 911) and the third link (early defibrillation). CPR allows oxygen to flow to the brain and heart until defibrillation or other advanced care can restore normal heart action. *Victims of out-of-hospital cardiac arrest who receive CPR by bystanders are more than twice as likely to survive as victims who do not receive such support.* The earlier you give CPR to a person in cardiac or respiratory arrest, the greater the victim's chance of survival.

Third Link: Early Defibrillation

Many adult victims of sudden cardiac arrest have **ventricular fibrillation (VF)**. VF is an abnormal, chaotic heart rhythm that prevents the heart from pumping blood.

The only treatment for VF is defibrillation. **Defibrillation** is a shock that stops VF and allows a normal heart rhythm to resume. When VF is present, prompt defibrillation will increase the victim's chance of survival. With each minute that defibrillation is delayed during cardiac arrest

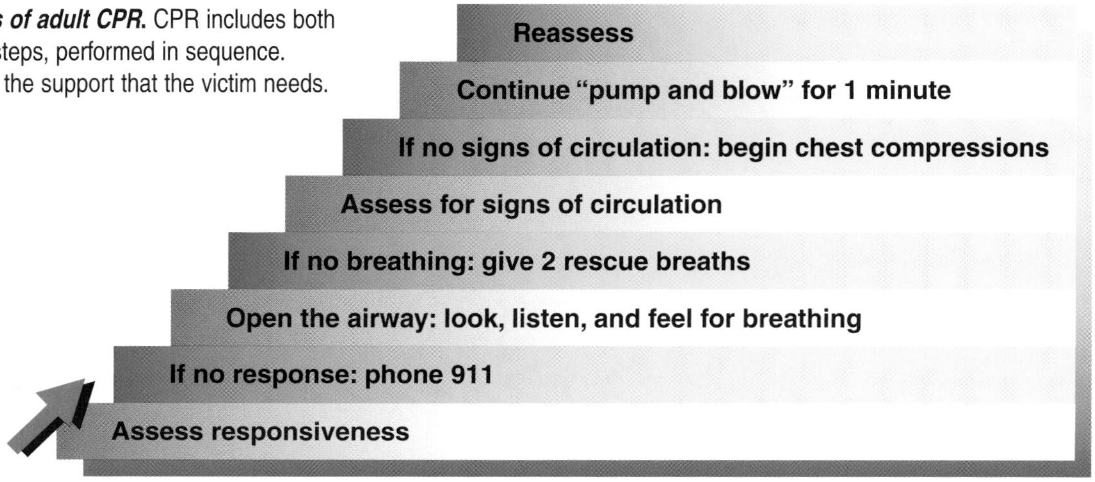

FIGURE 2. *The steps of adult CPR.* CPR includes both assessment and support steps, performed in sequence. The rescuer provides only the support that the victim needs.

Reassess

Continue "pump and blow" for 1 minute

If no signs of circulation: begin chest compressions

Assess for signs of circulation

If no breathing: give 2 rescue breaths

Open the airway: look, listen, and feel for breathing

If no response: phone 911

Assess responsiveness

FYI...

Automated External Defibrillators and Public Access Defibrillation Program

Automated external defibrillators (AEDs) are computerized defibrillators that may be safely operated by lay rescuers who have received a few hours of training. AEDs are extremely accurate and relatively inexpensive, and they can reduce the time to defibrillation if they are used before EMS personnel arrive. The AED is attached to the victim with 2 adhesive pads. The AED analyzes the electrical activity of the victim's heart and then determines if a shock is needed. The rescuer presses a SHOCK button to deliver the shock when prompted by the AED.

Public access defibrillation (PAD) is a public health initiative developed by the AHA. PAD programs are designed to increase the number of AEDs available in a community and the number of rescuers trained to provide CPR and use the defibrillators. In communities with PAD programs AEDs can be used by firefighters, police officers, airline personnel, and trained lay rescuers before EMS personnel arrive. When AEDs are used before the arrival of EMS personnel, they reduce the time to defibrillation and increase survival from out-of-hospital cardiac arrest.

You can be trained to provide CPR and operate an AED by taking the AHA Heartsaver AED Course. *Contact your local AHA for more details.*

caused by VF, the victim's chance of survival is reduced by 7% to 10%. If defibrillation is provided within the first 5 minutes of a VF cardiac arrest, the victim's chance of survival is about 50%. After 10 to 12 minutes of cardiac arrest there is very little chance of a successful rescue *unless CPR has been provided*. CPR prolongs the time that defibrillation can be effective, increasing the "window of opportunity" for resuscitation. To increase the victim's chance of survival, you must provide CPR until the defibrillator arrives.

In many locations throughout the United States, early community defibrillation programs, or *public access defibrillation* (PAD) programs, have been established. In PAD programs trained lay rescuers are equipped with AEDs. As noted above, if you provide CPR in a location served by a PAD program (for example, some golf courses or shopping malls), you (or the person who

phones 911) should get the AED and place it at the victim's side. When a rescuer trained in the use of AEDs arrives, early defibrillation can be performed without further delay.

Fourth Link: Advanced Care

The fourth link in the Chain of Survival is advanced care. Highly trained EMS personnel called *emergency medical technicians* (EMTs) provide CPR and defibrillation. Paramedics also provide CPR and defibrillation as well as more advanced care, such as use of cardiac drugs and breathing tubes. These advanced actions help the heart in VF to respond to defibrillation or maintain a normal rhythm after successful defibrillation. Advanced care is also provided in the hospital.

How to Recognize Life-Threatening Emergencies

- **Heart Attack**
- **Cardiac Arrest**
- **Stroke**
- **Choking**

How to Recognize a Heart Attack

Recall the case scenario of the father at the picnic on the beach who suddenly developed chest pain. He is pale, sweaty, and nauseated and complains of tightness in his chest that has lasted 10 minutes and has moved to his neck, jaw, and left arm. Are his symptoms consistent with the signs of a heart attack?

A heart attack means some heart muscle has suddenly started to die. The muscle is dying because one of the blood vessels of the heart (a coronary artery) has become blocked. New drugs called **clotbusters** can unblock the arteries of the heart if they are given within a few hours of the onset of signs of a heart attack. *Acute myocardial infarction* is the medical term for heart attack.

A person who is having a heart attack is usually awake and can talk to you but feels severe pain. The most critical time for treatment of a heart attack with clotbusters is within the first 90 minutes after symptoms begin. If you suspect someone is having a heart attack, activate the EMS system *immediately* (phone 911). These minutes count! Know the symptoms!

The most important and most common symptom of a heart attack is chest pain, discomfort, or pressure in the center of the chest, behind the breastbone (sternum). The pain may travel to the neck or jaw or down the left arm. It usually lasts more than 3 to 5 minutes. **Chest pain** is a *red flag.* The flag says **Warning! Think heart attack.**

Ask these questions:

- **"What is the pain like?"** People describe the pain of a heart attack in many ways: pressure, fullness, squeezing, or heaviness.

- **"Where is the pain located?"** People usually feel the pain right behind the breastbone, deep in the center of the chest **(see Figure 3)**. After a few moments the pain may spread to the shoulder, neck, or lower jaw or down the arm. The pain may be on the left side, right side, or both sides but is often on the left side. Sometimes the pain or discomfort may even be felt in the back, between the shoulder blades.

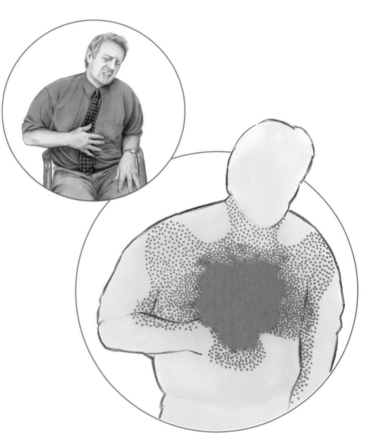

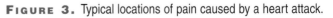

FIGURE 3. Typical locations of pain caused by a heart attack.

■ *"How long have you had the pain?"* The discomfort of a heart attack usually lasts more than a few minutes. Sharp, stabbing, knifelike pain that lasts only a second and then disappears is usually not the pain of a heart attack. But chest pain caused by a heart attack sometimes "stutters." This means the pain may stop completely and then return a short time later.

Not all warning symptoms occur in every heart attack. People who are having a heart attack may have vague signs. They may say they feel lightheaded, faint, short of breath, or nauseated, or they may describe their chest discomfort as an ache, heartburn, or indigestion. These vague signs of a heart attack are more common in women, people with diabetes, and the elderly.

Many people will not admit that they might be having a heart attack. People react with a variety of statements or excuses. They may say "I'm too

---

Critical Concepts

Most Common Warning Signs and Symptoms of Heart Attack

Not *all* warning symptoms occur in *every* heart attack. If *any* occur, don't wait. Get help immediately. Phone 911. Delay can be deadly! People who are having a heart attack may complain of signs or symptoms other than chest pain. The most common red flags, or warning symptoms, of a heart attack include

■ Uncomfortable pressure, fullness, squeezing or pain in the center of the chest

■ Pain that spreads to the shoulders, neck or arms.

■ Chest discomfort with lightheadedness, fainting, sweating, nausea or shortness of breath.

Critical Concepts

Remember the critical actions you should take if you are alone and find someone who is unresponsive:

■ Phone 911 (or other emergency response number) and get the AED if available.
■ Begin CPR.

---

healthy," or "I don't want to bother the doctor," or "I don't want to frighten my wife," or "I'll feel ridiculous if it isn't a heart attack," or "I hate red lights and sirens." When a person with symptoms of a heart attack tries to downplay what he or she is feeling, **you** must take responsibility and act at once. Tell the victim to sit quietly. Phone 911 or send someone to phone 911 and get the AED (if one is available). Be prepared to perform CPR.

You must phone 911 immediately for 2 reasons. First, EMS personnel can rapidly transport the victim to the hospital and provide medical care during transport. EMS personnel are prepared to treat potential complications of a heart attack, particularly abnormal heart rhythms and cardiac arrest. Second, EMS personnel can alert the hospital about the arrival of a patient with a potential heart attack. The hospital will then be better prepared to administer drugs such as clot-busters that may dissolve the clot and reduce or eliminate damage to the heart. These new drugs are effective only if they are given within the first few hours after the onset of symptoms of a heart attack. For these reasons, it is extremely important to phone 911.

After you phone 911, have the person rest quietly and calmly. Help the person into a position that is comfortable and that allows the easiest breathing.

How to Recognize a Cardiac Arrest

Recall the scenario used throughout this chapter. The father at the picnic complains of chest pain, which he says is caused by indigestion. He suddenly slumps over on the blanket and does not respond to voice or touch.

What should you do?

When an artery of the heart is blocked during a heart attack, the heart muscle is deprived of oxygen, and the heart may stop pumping blood. The heart muscle may quiver in the abnormal heart rhythm called ventricular fibrillation. This produces **cardiac arrest**—blood flow stops. Without blood flow to the brain, the person becomes unresponsive, collapses, stops breathing normally, and has no signs of circulation. The only treatment for VF is defibrillation with a defibrillator. If CPR is provided until the defibrillator arrives, defibrillation is more likely to be successful.

VF can develop as a complication of a heart attack, even in men or women who have no chest pain. In fact, VF and sudden cardiac arrest may be the *only* sign of a heart attack in some victims.

Sudden loss of responsiveness is a red flag. Act immediately! The victim may be in *cardiac arrest.* The **victim of cardiac arrest** will have **3 red flag signs:**

1. **No response:** Victims of cardiac arrest do not respond when you speak to them or touch them. If you are alone with someone who suddenly becomes unresponsive, immediately phone 911 or other emergency response number. If a second rescuer is present, send that rescuer to phone 911 (or other emergency response number) and get the AED if one is available while you begin CPR.

2. **No normal breathing:** Once you discover that the victim is unresponsive and 911 has been called, begin CPR. Open the airway and look, listen, and feel for breathing. The person in cardiac arrest does not take a normal breath when you check for breathing. You should then give the victim 2 rescue breaths.

3. **No signs of circulation:** After you provide 2 rescue breaths to the victim, check for signs of circulation. Look for a response from the victim to the initial breaths, such as normal breathing, coughing, or movement. If the heart is beating and delivering oxygen to the brain and body, the victim should react in some way after you deliver the 2 rescue breaths. Check for signs of circulation for no more than 10 seconds. If no signs of circulation are present, begin chest compressions. The steps of CPR are summarized in Chapter 2 of this module.

FYI...

Respiratory Arrest

Respiratory arrest is present when the victim is not breathing at all or is breathing so slowly, shallowly, or irregularly that oxygenation of the blood cannot occur. The term *respiratory arrest* is used for victims who are not breathing effectively but who still have signs of circulation. You can determine that respiratory arrest has occurred only when you go through the steps of CPR. A victim in respiratory arrest will be unresponsive. Open the airway and look, listen, and feel for breathing. You will see no breathing or only occasional or very shallow breathing effort. Give 2 breaths, watching the chest to see if it rises with each breath. The victim in respiratory arrest will show signs of circulation (breathing, coughing, or movement in response to the rescue breaths), confirming that the victim has spontaneous blood flow (circulation) and cardiac arrest is *not* present. However, the victim does not show normal, effective breathing, so respiratory arrest *is* present.

How to Recognize a Stroke

Recall the case scenario of the family having a picnic at the beach. The grandfather developed a headache and sudden signs of facial weakness and weakness on the right side of his body. Are these signs of a stroke?

What should you do?

Stroke is a leading cause of death and serious disability among Americans. A stroke is the rapid onset of neurologic problems, including weakness or paralysis of one or more limbs (particularly the arms), facial weakness, difficulty speaking, visual problems, intense dizziness, altered responsiveness, or severe headache. A stroke may occur when a blood vessel in the brain becomes blocked so that an area of the brain receives no blood flow and no oxygen. Or it can develop when a blood vessel in the brain ruptures and bleeds in the brain. Strokes are common and serious. Although most strokes occur in older people, *strokes can happen in people of all ages*.

Strokes occasionally cause damage in areas of the brain that control breathing, or the stroke may cause the victim to become unresponsive. If this occurs, the victim may stop breathing or develop airway obstruction. If these complications arise, you may need to perform some or all of the steps of CPR, particularly rescue breathing.

You must know the **signs of stroke** so that you can activate the EMS system. Unfortunately many signs of stroke are vague or are ignored by the victim. If you are concerned that someone has had a stroke, look closely for the sudden onset of one of these *red flags:*

1. **Facial droop:** This is most obvious if the victim smiles or grimaces. If one side of the face droops or the face does not move **(see Figure 4)**, a stroke may have occurred.

2. **Arm weakness:** This is most obvious if the victim extends his or her arms with the eyes closed **(see Figure 5)**. If one arm drifts downward or the victim cannot move his or her arms, a stroke may have occurred.

3. **Speech difficulties:** This is most obvious if the victim is unable to talk or slurs words. Ask the victim to repeat a sentence such as "You can't teach an old dog new tricks." If the victim cannot repeat the sentence accurately and clearly, a stroke may have occurred.

Whenever you think someone is having a stroke, phone 911 or other emergency response number!

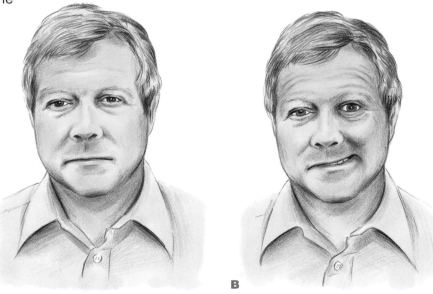

A   B

FIGURE 4. **A.** Normal. **B.** Facial droop in a stroke victim on the right side of the face.

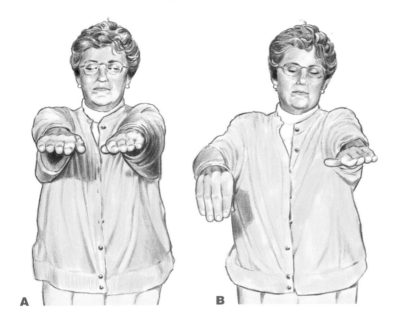

FIGURE 5. **A.** Normal. **B.** Arm weakness in a stroke victim.

EMS personnel will examine and quickly transport the victim to a hospital for evaluation and treatment.

New and effective treatments for stroke are now available, but they must be given *within the first 3 hours* after the onset of signs of a stroke. These drugs include clotbusters for the brain (fibrinolytic agents), that may reduce the disability caused by a stroke. Because the window of opportunity for administration of these new stroke treatments is narrow, the victim must get to a hospital *immediately*. EMS personnel can notify the hospital of the victim's condition before arrival to ensure that the victim receives rapid evaluation and therapy.

To help treat a stroke victim, it is essential that bystanders and lay rescuers

- Recognize the signs of stroke
- Phone 911 (or other emergency response number in your area)
- Provide CPR if needed

Family members and bystanders often fail to phone 911 when a stroke occurs. Do not make the mistake of thinking that the stroke victim's symptoms are caused by alcohol or drug intoxication or medical conditions such as low blood sugar. *If you suspect that a person is having a stroke, do not delay: Phone 911 or other emergency response number immediately.*

How to Recognize Choking

Every year choking (foreign-body airway obstruction) causes about 3000 deaths in the United States. Choking in adults usually occurs during eating. Meat is the most frequent cause of choking in adults, but a variety of foods and foreign bodies can obstruct the airway.

Foreign objects may *partially* block the airway but still allow adequate air movement. Choking victims with only *partial obstruction* of the airway will remain responsive and cough forcefully, and usually they can speak. Breath sounds may be noisy. These victims require no immediate action from you, but be prepared to act if the obstruction becomes severe or complete.

Victims with *severe or complete* airway obstruction will remain responsive at first but will not be able to move enough air to cough forcefully or speak. They may make high-pitched noises when they try to inhale. You must be prepared to help relieve the obstruction with abdominal thrusts (the Heimlich maneuver).

You do **not** need to act if the victim can cough forcefully and speak. A victim who can cough and speak has only a partially blocked airway and is able to move air. **Do not interfere** at this point because a strong cough is the most effective way to remove a foreign object. Stay with the victim and monitor his or her condition. If the choking persists, phone 911.

To treat airway obstruction successfully, **you must first recognize it.** If a foreign object is completely blocking the airway, remove it. Review the adjacent box and the list below to remember the *red flag* signs of severe choking:

- Universal choking sign **(see Figure 6)**
- Victim unable to speak (ask the victim, "Are you choking?" If the victim nods, ask, "Can you speak?")
- Weak, ineffective coughs
- High-pitched sounds or no sounds while inhaling
- Increased difficulty breathing
- Blue lips or skin (cyanosis)

Causes and Prevention of Choking

The best way to treat choking is to **prevent it from happening in the first place.** Factors that contribute to choking in adults include

- Swallowing large, poorly chewed pieces of food
- Eating while blood alcohol levels are elevated
- Wearing dentures
- Playing, crying, laughing, or talking with food or foreign objects in the mouth

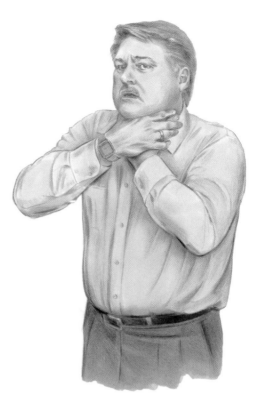

FIGURE 6. Universal choking sign (hands clutching the throat).

Critical Concepts

Warning Signs of Severe Choking

- Universal sign of choking — victim is clutching the neck with one or both hands **(see Figure 6)**
- Ask the victim, "Are you choking?" If the victim nods, ask, "Can you speak?" If the victim is **unable to speak** or has any of the signs listed below, perform abdominal thrusts (Heimlich maneuver).
- Weak, ineffective coughs
- High-pitched sounds or no sounds while inhaling
- Increased difficulty breathing
- Blue lips or skin (cyanosis)

Choking may be prevented by

- Cutting food into small pieces and chewing slowly and thoroughly, especially if you wear dentures
- Avoiding excessive intake of alcohol, particularly while eating
- Avoiding laughing and talking while chewing and swallowing

Foundation Facts

Causes of Airway Obstruction

There are 3 common ways in which an adult's airway may become obstructed. Each is treated differently.

1. **Foreign body.** A foreign object (for example, food) may become lodged in the air passage, blocking the airway. If an adult develops signs of choking, give abdominal thrusts (the Heimlich maneuver) until the object is expelled or the victim becomes unresponsive.

2. **Relaxed tongue.** In an unresponsive victim (for example, after a stroke or head injury or during cardiac arrest), the tongue may fall back against the throat, blocking the airway. Use either the head tilt–chin lift maneuver or the jaw-thrust technique described in Chapter 2 to lift the tongue away from the back of the throat.

3. **Swollen air passages.** This condition is a *medical* problem caused by an infection or inflammation, not a *mechanical* problem caused by a foreign object. Medications are needed to treat swollen air passages, and the victim may need help breathing. Abdominal thrusts or other CPR techniques will *not* relieve this type of airway obstruction.

Protecting Your Heart and Blood Vessels

The blood vessels in your heart and brain require special care to remain healthy and clear of obstructions. Cigarette smoking, high blood pressure, a diet high in fat, and other factors can damage blood vessels and obstruct blood flow. If your blood vessels are damaged or obstructed, they can gradually narrow, and blood clots can form, resulting in a heart attack or stroke.

The Table on the next page lists the major controllable risk factors for heart attack and stroke. Take a moment to review these risk factors and lifestyle changes needed to achieve a healthy lifestyle.

Other risk factors for heart attack and stroke include heredity, being male, increasing age, diabetes, stress, and race (African Americans have the greatest risk of heart attack and stroke). Contact your local AHA for more information on preventing heart attack and stroke or visit the AHA website at www.americanheart.org.

Major Controllable Risk Factors for Heart Attack and Stroke

Factor	Explanation	Lifestyle Behavior to Reduce Risk
Cigarette Smoking	Cigarette smoking is the most important single cause of preventable death in the United States. Smoking and second-hand smoke can damage blood vessels and cause many other preventable diseases. Second-hand smoke can also hurt your loved ones.	Stop smoking as soon as possible. Pick a day *now* to quit. Ask your doctor for help. The greatest gift you can give yourself, your loved ones, and your friends is to quit smoking.
High Blood Pressure	Uncontrolled high blood pressure increases your risk of heart attack and stroke. High blood pressure can damage the blood vessels, including those in the brain.	Have your blood pressure checked frequently. If you have high blood pressure, see your doctor, and take your prescribed medications as instructed.
High Blood Cholesterol	Excess cholesterol can be deposited on the inner walls of the arteries, narrowing them. This can reduce blood flow to the heart or brain.	Have your doctor check your blood cholesterol levels regularly. Avoid a diet high in saturated fat.
Lack of Exercise	Lack of exercise can contribute to factors that can cause a heart attack. However, vigorous exercise by persons who have not exercised regularly can be dangerous. Talk to your doctor before you start an exercise program.	With your doctor's help, plan a regular exercise program and stick to it.
Obesity	Obesity increases the risk of high blood pressure, diabetes, and high blood cholesterol, all of which increase the risk of heart attack and stroke.	Develop a healthy diet with help from your doctor. Fad diets do not produce long-term weight loss.
Heart Disease	Heart disease is a major risk factor for heart attack and stroke.	Follow your doctor's advice for treating heart disease.
Transient Ischemic Attacks (TIAs)	TIAs are strokelike symptoms that disappear in less than 24 hours. TIAs are strong predictors of stroke. They are usually treated with drugs that keep blood clots from forming.	If stroke symptoms occur, phone 911 or other emergency response number and seek immediate evaluation in the nearest Emergency Department.

Summary

To rescue someone you must first recognize that the person is having an emergency. The Chain of Survival for heart attack, cardiac arrest, stroke, and choking starts with YOU, someone who is trained to recognize the emergency and take action. Recognizing warning signs is an important step that will be practiced in this course.

This course encourages each participant to become a part of the community's Chain of Survival:

- Learn to recognize 4 conditions that are major killers in the United States: heart attack, cardiac arrest, stroke, and choking.
- Know to phone 911 or other emergency response number in your area for these emergencies.
- Know how to perform CPR.

With this knowledge and these skills you can become an effective and vital link in your community's Chain of Survival.

Learning Checklist

Take a moment to review the key information you have learned in this chapter before evaluating your knowledge.

- The 4 links in the adult Chain of Survival are
  - Phone 911 or other emergency response number (and get the AED if available)
  - CPR
  - Early defibrillation
  - Advanced care
- Early defibrillation is needed to treat VF. The sooner defibrillation is attempted, the better the victim's chance of survival.

- AEDs can be operated by trained laypersons, such as those who have completed the AHA Heartsaver AED Course. When defibrillation is provided within the first few minutes after collapse, the victim's chance of surviving a cardiac arrest caused by VF is greatly improved.
- The signs and symptoms of heart attack:
  - The most common symptom of a heart attack is pain, pressure, squeezing, or heaviness in the center of the chest behind the breastbone (sternum) that may travel to the neck or jaw or down the left arm.
  - Many people (particularly women, people with diabetes, and the elderly) have vague signs and symptoms of a heart attack, such as sweaty skin, lightheadedness, fainting, shortness of breath, or nausea and discomfort described as an ache, heartburn, or indigestion.
- Three *red flags* of cardiac arrest are
  - No response
  - No normal breathing
  - No signs of circulation
- Three *red flags* of stroke are
  - Facial droop
  - Arm weakness
  - Speech difficulties
- The red flags of severe or complete foreign-body airway obstruction are
  - Universal sign of choking (the victim clutches his or her neck)
  - Inability to speak (ask, "Can you speak?")
  - Weak, ineffective coughs
  - High-pitched or no sounds while inhaling
  - Increased difficulty breathing
  - Blue lips or skin (cyanosis)

Review Questions

1. **You are alone and you discover your 64-year-old friend lying unresponsive on the floor. What do you do next?**

   a. phone 911 or other emergency response number
   b. begin CPR
   c. perform rescue breathing
   d. transfer to advanced care

2. **During a game of basketball your father stops playing and then becomes pale and sweaty and complains of chest discomfort. You suspect he is having a heart attack. Which of the following is a *red flag* warning sign of heart attack that should prompt you to phone 911?**

   a. squeezing or crushing chest pain behind the breastbone that lasts more than a few minutes
   b. sharp, stabbing chest pain that lasts only a few seconds
   c. shortness of breath
   d. a headache your father describes as "the worst headache of my life"

3. **At the supermarket an elderly man suddenly clutches his chest and collapses. You go to his aid, find that he is unresponsive, and ask a bystander to phone 911. Which of the following groups of signs or symptoms are the *red flag* warning signs of cardiac arrest?**

   a. facial droop, arm weakness, and speech difficulties
   b. chest pain, lightheadedness, sweating, and nausea
   c. no response, no normal breathing, and no signs of circulation
   d. no response, spontaneous breathing, and chest pain

4. **You are talking with your supervisor when she begins to slur her words. You suspect she is having a stroke. Which of the following signs or symptoms are the *red flag* warning signs of stroke that should prompt you to phone 911 or other emergency response number?**

   a. sudden loss of responsiveness and cardiac arrest
   b. facial droop, arm weakness, and speech difficulties
   c. no response, no normal breathing, and no signs of circulation
   d. crushing chest pain that lasts a few minutes, nausea, and sweating

5. **A 22-year-old woman engaged in conversation at the table next to yours in the cafeteria suddenly begins to cough forcefully and then clutches her neck and becomes silent. Which of the following signs or symptoms are the *red flag* warning signs of severe choking that prompt you to perform the Heimlich maneuver?**

   a. hoarse speech and wheezing between coughs
   b. severe, forceful coughing
   c. inability to speak, breathe, or cough forcefully and blue skin or lips
   d. no response, no normal breathing, and no signs of circulation

How did you do?

1, a; **2,** a; **3,** c; **4,** b; **5,** c.

Module 1

Chapter **2** *The ABCs of CPR*
Techniques of Adult CPR

Case Scenario

You were walking on the beach, and you visited briefly with a family on a picnic. The family consisted of a grandfather, a father, a child, and an infant. You return to the area in response to a shout for help. You find the father clutching his chest, looking pale, and complaining of crushing chest pain that has lasted 10 minutes and has now spread to his jaw and right arm. He denies that he could be having a heart attack, and he asks for antacids. Suddenly he falls to the ground and does not move or respond when touched.

Do you know what to do?

In this chapter you will learn the steps of CPR. You begin the steps of CPR when you find an unresponsive adult victim.

Learning Objectives

After reading this chapter, you should be able to

1. Recognize cardiac arrest
2. Describe and demonstrate phoning 911 (or other emergency response number), rescue breathing using the mouth-to-mouth and mouth-to-barrier techniques, and 1-rescuer CPR
3. Recognize when someone is choking as a result of a foreign-body airway obstruction
4. Describe and demonstrate how to clear a foreign-body airway obstruction in a responsive person

CPR: The Second Link in the Adult Chain of Survival

CPR, the second link in the adult Chain of Survival, is a set of assessments and skills used in sequence to provide rescue support and maintain some oxygen and blood flow to the heart and brain. CPR skills include a combination of rescue breathing (blowing), which you provide if the victim is not breathing, and chest compressions (pumping), which you perform if the victim has no signs of circulation.

CPR helps the victim even if ventricular fibrillation is present because CPR helps the heart respond better to defibrillation attempts. You must begin CPR at once to provide oxygen to the heart and increase the chance that defibrillation will succeed.

If you find an *unresponsive person* and other rescuers are available, send someone to **phone 911 or other emergency response number** (and get an AED if available). ***Then YOU start CPR.*** Continue CPR until additional treatment (defibrillation) restores normal heart action or until EMS personnel arrive. If you are alone, phone 911 or other emergency response number (and get the AED if available) and then return to the victim to begin CPR.

Critical Concepts

Unresponsive? Phone 911 and get the AED (if available)

To help remember these first actions, think of this short phrase: **Unresponsive? Phone 911 and get the AED.**

You must be sure that you or another person takes these actions. Then begin CPR.

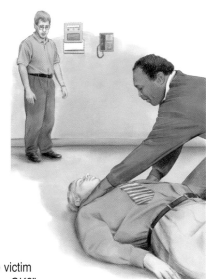

FIGURE 7.
Check for response
by gently shaking the victim
and shouting, "Are you OK?"

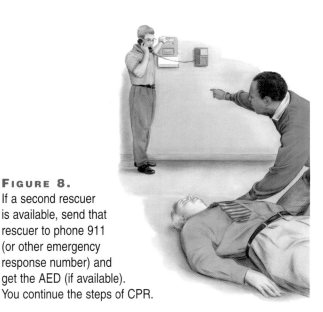

FIGURE 8.
If a second rescuer
is available, send that
rescuer to phone 911
(or other emergency
response number) and
get the AED (if available).
You continue the steps of CPR.

The assessment and skills steps of CPR are simple.

1. **Check response: Check whether the victim is responsive** by gently shaking the victim and shouting, "Are you OK?" **(see Figure 7)**.

   - **If the victim is *unresponsive,* phone 911 or send someone to phone 911 (or other emergency response number)** and get an AED if available. The call to 911 activates the EMS system and ensures that professional help is on the way. The AHA recommends that in out-of-hospital settings AEDs be stored next to the telephone to ensure rapid access to both 911 and the AED **(see Figure 8).**

   - **If you are alone** and find an unresponsive victim, leave the victim to phone 911 and get an AED if available.

   - When you or someone else has phoned 911, kneel at the victim's side near his head to start CPR. Carefully turn the victim onto his back if needed. If you suspect the victim is injured, turn the head, neck, and body as one unit.

2. **Airway: Open the airway (see Figures 9 and 10).**

   - *Head tilt–chin lift:* Tilt the head back by lifting the chin gently with one hand while pushing down on the forehead with the other hand **(see Figure 9).**

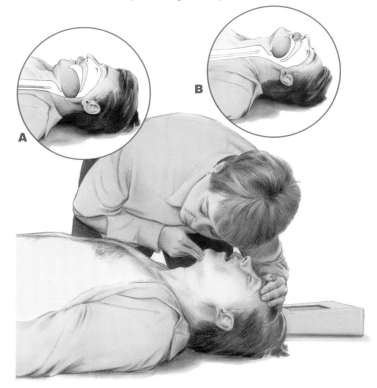

FIGURE 9. Open the airway with the head tilt–chin lift technique. **A.** In an unresponsive victim, the tongue falls back to obstruct the airway. **B.** The head tilt–chin lift technique lifts the tongue away from the back of the throat and opens the airway.

- *Jaw thrust:* If the victim has a possible injury to the head or neck, use the *jaw thrust* **(see Figure 10)** to open the airway. Lift the angles of the jaw. This moves the jaw and tongue forward and opens the airway without bending the neck.

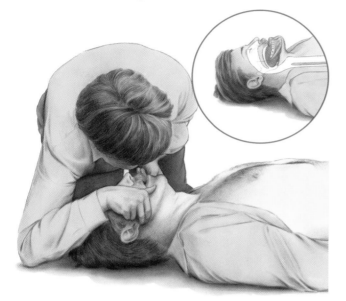

FIGURE 10. Open the airway by using the jaw-thrust technique. Lifting on the angles of the jaw moves the jaw and tongue forward and opens the airway without bending the neck. Use the jaw thrust to open the airway when a head or neck injury may be present.

3. **Breathing: Hold the airway open and look, listen, and feel to determine if the victim is breathing normally (see Figure 11). If the victim is not breathing normally, provide rescue breaths.**

   To check for normal breathing, *look, listen,* and *feel for breathing:*
   a. Place your ear next to the victim's mouth and nose and listen for sounds of normal breathing, turning your head to look at the chest.
   b. Look for the chest to rise. Listen and feel for air movement on your cheek.

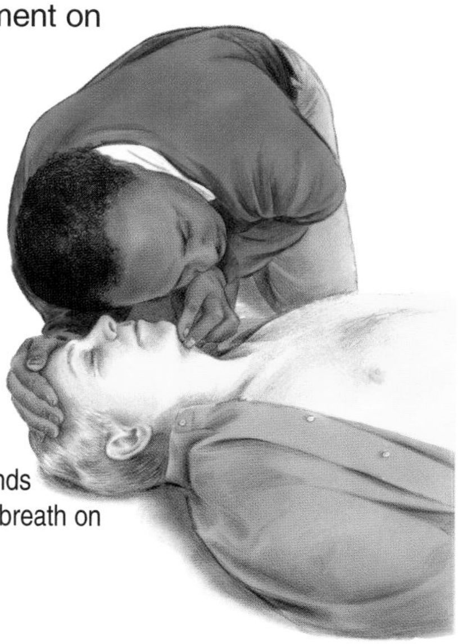

FIGURE 11. Place your ear next to the victim's mouth and nose and look at the victim's chest. *Look* for chest movement, *listen* for sounds of breathing, and *feel* for breath on your cheek.

FYI...

Opening the Airway With the Jaw Thrust

In CPR your first action is to open the **airway.** When the victim is unresponsive, the muscles of the jaw and neck relax, allowing the tongue to fall back against the throat and block the airway **(see Figure 9 A).** The **tongue** is the **most common cause** of a blocked airway in an unresponsive victim.

The tongue is attached to the lower jaw. There are 2 techniques to pull the tongue away from the back of the throat and open the airway: the head tilt–chin lift and the jaw thrust.

If you suspect that the victim has head or neck trauma, use only the *jaw thrust* to open the airway **(see Figure 10).** *Do not use the head tilt because it may worsen injury to the spinal cord.*

To perform the jaw thrust, grasp the angles of the victim's jaw (the portion of the jaw right below the earlobes) and lift the jaw *without* tilting the head. This method of opening the airway will pull the tongue away from the back of the throat without moving the head or neck. Use the jaw-thrust technique when you think the victim may have a head or neck injury.

The head tilt–chin lift method of airway opening is the technique you will be most likely to use, so it is emphasized in this course. Your instructor will demonstrate the jaw thrust and you should practice it with a manikin, but you will not be expected to demonstrate the jaw thrust during the skills demonstration at the end of the course.

If the victim is not breathing normally, give rescue breaths (see Figure 12).

To give rescue breaths,

a. Place your mouth around the victim's mouth and pinch the nose closed **(see Figure 12A).**

b. Continue to tilt the head and lift the chin (or perform the jaw thrust).

c. Give 2 slow breaths (approximately 2 seconds each).

d. Be sure the victim's chest rises each time you give a rescue breath. If the chest does not rise when you give a rescue breath, reopen the airway (using head tilt–chin lift) and try to give the rescue breaths again.

e. If a barrier device is available for CPR in the workplace, use the barrier device **(see Figure 12B)** to provide rescue breathing (see "Barrier Devices and Masks" later in this chapter).

4. **Circulation:** After you deliver 2 rescue breaths, look for signs of circulation:

a. Look for any response to the 2 rescue breaths. The victim may start breathing normally, coughing, or moving (see box below).

b. Do not take more than 10 seconds to check for signs of circulation.

c. If you are not confident that signs of circulation are present, start chest compressions.

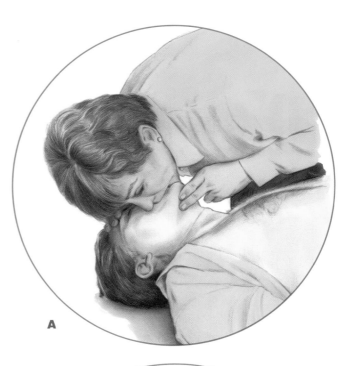

A

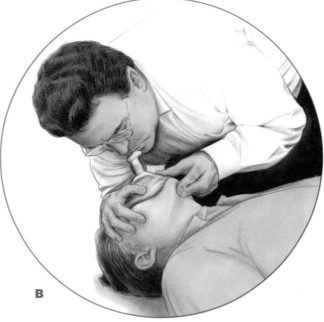

B

FIGURE 12. Rescue breathing. **A.** Mouth-to-mouth breathing. **B.** Mouth-to–barrier device breathing.

Critical Concepts

Check for Signs of Circulation

Blood must circulate to deliver oxygen to the brain, heart, and other vital organs. If you can identify signs of normal breathing, coughing, or movement, the victim's heart is beating adequately to supply blood to the body, and chest compressions are unnecessary. If you are not confident that signs of circulation are present, begin chest compressions.

Note: If the victim has signs of circulation, chest compressions are *not* required. If the victim is not breathing normally but signs of circulation *are* present, the victim is in **respiratory arrest** and you must continue to give rescue breaths (1 breath every 5 seconds).

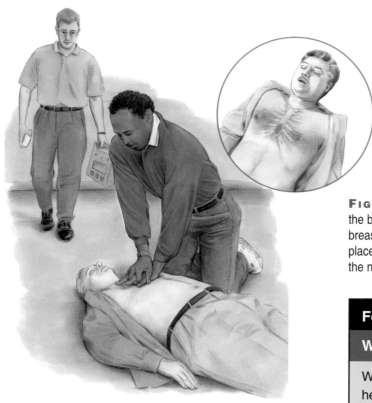

d. To provide chest compressions, place the heel of one hand on the center of the chest right between the nipples. This positions the hand on the lower half of the breastbone **(see Figure 13).**

e. Place the heel of the second hand on top of the first hand.

FIGURE 13. The rescuer compresses the lower half of the breastbone, being careful to avoid the very bottom of the breastbone. To find the proper location for chest compressions, place the heel of one hand in the center of the chest between the nipples.

Foundation Facts

Agonal Breathing and Respiratory Arrest

People in cardiac arrest soon stop breathing. Some victims may display irregular, infrequent, gasping breaths called "agonal breaths." Agonal breaths may fool some rescuers into thinking that the victim is still alive, still breathing, and not in need of rescue breathing or other steps of CPR. This could mean that you will miss an opportunity to save a person's life.

If the victim is unresponsive and is not breathing *normally,* provide 2 rescue breaths and be sure that the chest rises with each breath. If the victim has no signs of circulation (no breathing, coughing, or movement in response to the 2 rescue breaths), the victim is in cardiac arrest.

A victim in **respiratory arrest** is unresponsive and is not breathing normally but has signs of circulation. This victim requires rescue breathing but not chest compressions. A victim in **cardiac arrest** is unresponsive, is not breathing normally, and has no signs of circulation. This victim requires all the steps of CPR (compressions and ventilations).

Foundation Facts

Why Is Rescue Breathing Important?

When breathing stops, delivery of oxygen to the heart and brain stops. If delivery of oxygen is not restored quickly, the heart and brain may be damaged. The longer the victim is deprived of oxygen, the smaller the chance that he or she will respond to CPR. Even if CPR is effective, it may take several minutes for a victim to begin breathing again. Mouth-to-mouth breathing is the fastest way to deliver oxygen to the victim's lungs and blood.

When providing rescue breathing, check to see that the victim's chest rises with each breath you give. This is critical because it is the only way you can be sure that you are giving good rescue breaths. If the chest does not rise when you deliver the breaths, reopen the airway (with head tilt–chin lift) and reattempt to deliver the breaths.

You must deliver rescue breaths *slowly.* Take 2 seconds to deliver each breath. *Do not* give rapid, forceful breaths because you will blow air into the esophagus and stomach instead of the lungs. Air in the stomach can cause vomiting, which complicates CPR in many ways. Too much air in the lungs can also be damaging.

If a victim has dentures, leave them in place unless they are extremely loose. Dentures help provide a good mouth-to-mouth seal. Remove loose dentures because they do not help you make a good mouth-to-mouth seal and they may fall back into the throat and obstruct the airway.

f. Position your body directly over your hands. Your shoulders should be above your hands, your elbows should be straight (not bent), and you should look down on your hands.

g. Provide 15 compressions at a rate of about 100 per minute. (**Note:** The rate of compressions is slightly less than 2 compressions per second. You will actually deliver less than 100 compressions per minute because you will stop compressions to provide rescue breaths.)

    ■ Push the breastbone in (compress) 1½ to 2 inches with each compression.

    ■ Allow the chest to relax (return to its normal shape) between compressions, but leave your hands on the chest between compressions (do not lift your hands off the chest).

5. **"Pump and blow": Provide cycles of 15 chest compressions and 2 rescue breaths.**

    a. Continue CPR with 15 chest compressions (pump) and 2 slow breaths (blow).

    b. After approximately 1 minute of CPR (about 4 cycles of 15 compressions and 2 breaths), check for signs of circulation. Check for signs of circulation every few minutes. If signs of circulation return, stop chest compressions and continue to provide rescue breathing as needed (1 breath every 5 seconds).

6. **Recovery Position:** If the victim develops signs of circulation, chest compressions are no longer necessary. If the victim resumes normal breathing, it is no longer necessary to provide rescue breathing. Place the victim in a position that will hold the airway open and continue to monitor the victim's breathing. If there are no signs of trauma, turn the victim onto his side in the recovery position **(see Figure 14).** If trauma has occurred, leave the victim on his back and hold the airway open using a jaw thrust as needed.

FYI...

Difference Between Compression Rate and Number of Compressions *Actually Delivered* per Minute

During adult CPR you compress the sternum at a rate of *approximately 100 times per minute*. This corresponds to a rate slightly less than 2 compressions per second during the groups of 15 compressions, so it won't take very many seconds to perform each set of 15 compressions. The term *compression rate* refers to the *speed* of compressions, not to the actual number of compressions *delivered* per minute. Note that this compression rate will actually provide less than 100 compressions each minute because you will pause to provide breaths after every 15 compressions. The actual number of compressions delivered per minute will vary from rescuer to rescuer and will be influenced by the compression rate and the speed with which you can position the head, open the airway, and deliver rescue breaths.

FYI...

Two-Rescuer CPR

CPR can also be performed by 2 rescuers. One rescuer assesses the victim and provides rescue breathing. The other rescuer gives chest compressions. Use the same ratio of chest compressions and rescue breaths used in 1-rescuer CPR: 15 compressions and 2 ventilations in each cycle.

Two-rescuer CPR may be taught as a module of the Heartsaver CPR Course. Your instructor will provide a 2-rescuer CPR performance sheet if needed in your course.

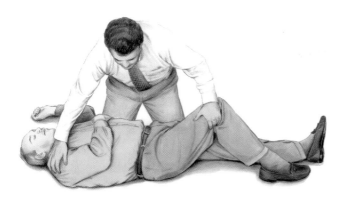

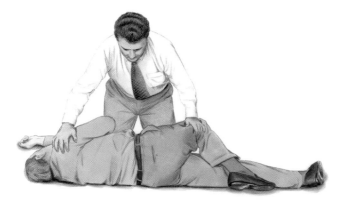

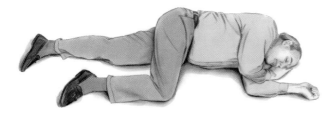

Figure 14. Recovery position. Several possible recovery positions can be used. The position should support the head and neck in a neutral position and should not place stress on joints or exert pressure over bony prominences.

Barrier Devices and Masks

Mouth-to-mouth rescue breathing may be life-saving for victims and is safe for rescuers. When you perform CPR you have almost no chance of becoming infected with viruses such as human immunodeficiency virus (HIV), the virus that causes AIDS, or any of the hepatitis viruses. To date no human has ever contracted HIV or hepatitis through mouth-to-mouth contact during CPR.

Some potential rescuers may hesitate to perform mouth-to-mouth rescue breathing because of concerns about infectious diseases. It is important to remember that approximately 70% of CPR is performed in the home or for a loved one or friend.

The AHA recommends the use of barrier devices to encourage bystanders to start CPR if they are concerned about mouth-to-mouth contact with the victim. The Occupational Safety and Health Administration recommends that barrier devices be available in the workplace and that employees who perform CPR in the workplace (for example, security guards and shopping mall employees) use barrier devices to prevent the spread of infection. However, a barrier device is not *required* to provide CPR.

Do *not* withhold rescue breathing from a victim of cardiac or respiratory arrest just because a barrier device is not immediately available. If you waste time trying to locate a device and remember how to use it, you may reduce the victim's chance of survival.

Regardless of whether a barrier device is available, the key actions of the rescuer remain the same: (1) Open the airway using the head tilt–chin lift maneuver (or jaw thrust if the victim has head or neck injuries), and (2) provide rescue breaths over about 2 seconds. When using a barrier device, position the face shield or mask securely over the victim's mouth, ensuring an adequate air seal. *Rescue breathing should be delivered through the barrier device with a force sufficient to make the chest rise.*

There are 2 types of barrier devices, face shields and face masks. In the Heartsaver CPR Adult Course you will learn about the barrier device that you will use during actual rescue breathing and CPR. Correct use requires practice. Practice on a manikin several times. The most critical step in using a face shield or mask is achieving a good seal around the mouth and nose because this prevents leakage of air during rescue breaths.

Face Shields

Face shields are clear plastic or silicon sheets that you place over the victim's face to keep your mouth from directly touching the victim. All face shields have an opening or tube in the center of the plastic sheet. This allows your rescue breaths to enter the victim's mouth. Face shields are small, flexible, and portable. A folded shield will fit easily in a packet on a key ring. If you keep the packet on your key ring, it is much more likely to be available when you need it.

Using a Face Shield

Remove the face shield from its plastic container or bag and unfold it. To use a face shield **(see Figure 15):**

- Position the face shield with the opening or tube over the victim's mouth, with the plastic covering the victim's nose also.
- Perform head tilt–chin lift.
- Place your mouth over the opening or tube in the face shield and provide slow rescue breaths (1 breath every 2 seconds) while watching the chest for movement.

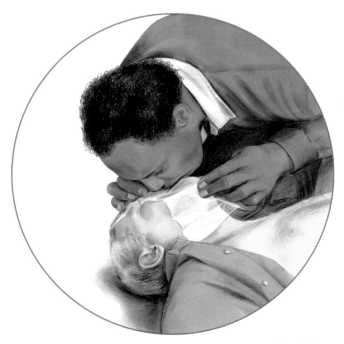

FIGURE 15. Rescuer preparing to perform rescue breathing with a face shield in place. Note that during rescue breathing the rescuer must ensure that the chest rises with each breath.

Face Masks

Face masks are firmer, more rigid devices that fit over the victim's mouth and nose. Masks are much easier to use than face shields, but they are bulkier, they cost more, and they are more inconvenient to carry around **(see Figure 16A).** This makes them less likely to be available if you unexpectedly need to perform CPR. Most face masks have 1-way valves that provide an effective barrier to movement of bacteria or viruses between the victim and rescuer.

Using a Face Mask

Most face masks are stored in a plastic container or bag. Some masks must be assembled before they can be used to provide rescue breathing. Become familiar with the face mask you will use *before* you need to use it in an emergency. You should be able to assemble the device within seconds.

To use a face mask, position yourself to the side of the victim's head in a location that will enable you to perform both rescue breathing and chest compressions and do the following **(see Figure 16B):**

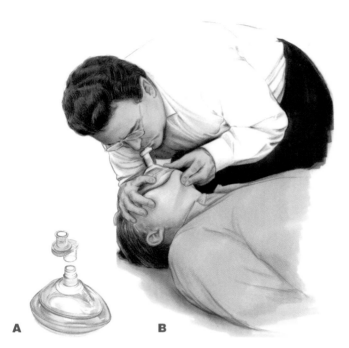

FIGURE 16. **A.** Face mask. **B.** Face mask held in place during rescue breathing. The face mask is held firmly against the face while the rescuer holds the airway open with head tilt–chin lift.

- Place the mask on the victim's face, using the bridge of the nose as a guide for correct position.
- Seal the mask by placing the index and thumb of your hand closest to the top of the victim's head along the border of the mask and placing the thumb of your other hand along the lower margin of the mask.
- Place the remaining fingers of your hand closest to the victim's feet along the bony margin of the jaw and lift the jaw while performing a head tilt **(see Figure 9B).**
- Compress firmly completely around the outside margin of the mask to provide a tight seal.
- Provide slow rescue breaths. Be sure that the chest rises with each breath.

Choking: Foreign-Body Airway Obstruction

Recall the case scenario presented earlier in this module. You have been called to help with an emergency on the beach. When you arrive at the scene, you see a father standing holding his throat with both hands, not speaking. The grandfather says, "I don't know what happened. He was eating chicken and suddenly coughed and then couldn't speak." You approach the father and say, "I know CPR — I can help you. Are you choking?" He nods. You then ask, "Can you speak?" He shakes his head and points to his throat. His lips are blue and he is making only very weak coughing sounds.

What should you do now?

Choking is an alarming and dramatic emergency. The desperate efforts of the choking person to clear his or her airway heighten the emotional drama and increase the pressure on the rescuer to take the correct action.

First Aid for Severe or Complete Airway Obstruction

Use the **Heimlich maneuver** (abdominal thrusts) to relieve severe or complete obstruction of the airway caused by a foreign object. Victims with severe or complete airway obstruction will not be able to cough forcefully or speak.

The Heimlich maneuver quickly forces air from the victim's lungs. This expels the blocking object like a cork from a bottle. Repeat abdominal thrusts until the object is expelled or the victim becomes unresponsive.

If the choking victim is *responsive* and *standing,* perform the Heimlich maneuver (see Figure 17):

1. Make a fist with one hand.
2. Place the thumb side of the fist on the victim's abdomen, slightly above the navel and well below the breastbone.
3. Grasp the fist with the other hand and provide quick upward thrusts into the victim's abdomen **(see Figure 17).**
4. Repeat the thrusts and continue until the object is expelled or the victim becomes unresponsive.

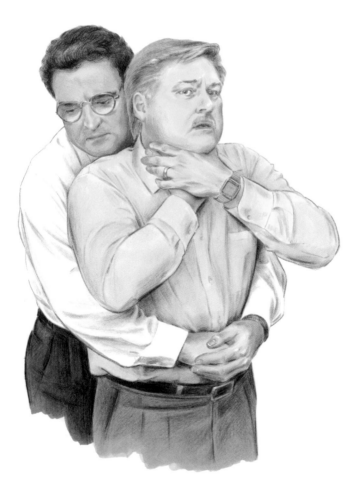

FIGURE 17. Heimlich maneuver for responsive victim with foreign-body airway obstruction. The rescuer stands behind victim, placing the fist of one hand on the victim's abdomen, slightly above the navel but below the breastbone, and grasps that fist with the other hand. The rescuer uses both hands to deliver quick upward thrusts until the object is expelled or the victim becomes unresponsive.

If severe or complete foreign-body airway obstruction is not relieved, the victim will stop breathing. Then the brain and heart will lack oxygen-rich blood. The victim will become unresponsive. When the victim becomes unresponsive and you are alone, **activate the EMS system by phoning 911 or other emergency response number** (*and get an AED if available*). Then attempt CPR. If someone else is present, send that person to phone 911 while you begin CPR.

There are 2 reasons why CPR may be effective for the person who becomes unresponsive from choking. First, when a victim becomes unresponsive, the muscles of the upper airway relax, and a *complete* airway obstruction may become an *incomplete* obstruction. If this happens, you may be able to deliver rescue breaths successfully past an incomplete obstruction. Second, evidence indicates that chest compressions may help relieve choking.

The steps you use to provide CPR for the victim who has become unresponsive after choking are the same as those described earlier in this chapter with one addition. When you open the airway to check for breathing and every time you open the airway to provide rescue breaths, open the mouth widely and look for a foreign body. If you see an object in the throat, remove it. Do not, however, spend a lot of time looking, and do not perform blind finger sweeps. If you do not see an object, continue the steps of CPR.

FYI...

First Aid for Choking in Pregnant and Obese Victims

If the choking victim is in the late stages of pregnancy or is obese, use chest thrusts instead of abdominal thrusts **(see Figure 18).** Stand behind the victim and wrap your arms around her. Position your hands (one in a fist, the other grasping it) on the chest on the center of the breastbone, between the nipples, and deliver sets of 5 chest thrusts until the object is expelled or the victim becomes unresponsive.

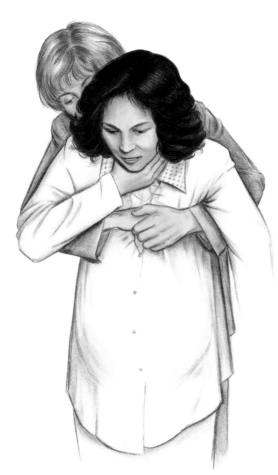

FIGURE 18. Chest thrusts administered to a conscious victim of foreign-body airway obstruction.

Keeping Your Skills Sharp: CPR Practice

Review the steps and skills of 1-rescuer CPR regularly (several times every year). If you learn CPR for a loved one at home, you can review the steps of CPR with practice videos and CPR prompt devices that use recorded instructions. Renew your CPR skills with an instructor at least every 2 years by taking an AHA renewal course.

Never rehearse or practice CPR skills on another person. Chest compressions can be lifesaving for a victim of cardiac arrest, but they can injure a responsive, healthy person.

Summary

The ABCs of CPR are an important set of skills that everyone should learn. In your lifetime you will probably encounter at least one emergency in which your ability to perform CPR will help save a life or prevent an urgent problem from becoming a life-threatening emergency.

A: **A**irway problems are common. Everyone should know the steps to take to

- Open the airway of an unresponsive victim (head tilt–chin lift or jaw thrust)
- Rescue a responsive choking victim with complete foreign-body airway obstruction (abdominal thrusts)

B: **B**reathing problems can occur during these emergencies:

- Respiratory and cardiac arrest
- Choking caused by a foreign body in the airway
- Strokes and seizures
- Head trauma
- Drowning and submersion (near-drowning)
- Medication overdoses and drug intoxication

To manage breathing problems, you must know how to open the airway and give rescue breaths.

C: **C**irculation problems may be present. You should support the circulation with *chest compressions* if the victim has no signs of circulation. The victim of cardiac arrest is unresponsive, is not breathing normally, and has no signs of circulation in response to rescue breaths.

The most common cause of sudden adult cardiac arrest is VF. Chest compressions are simple and easy to learn and will "buy time" until defibrillation is performed.

Learning Checklist

Take a moment to review the key information you have learned in this chapter before evaluating your knowledge.

✔ When you encounter an unresponsive victim, the steps for assessment and action are

- Phone 911 or other emergency response number (and get the AED if available).
- Open the airway and assess breathing.
- Give 2 slow rescue breaths if the victim is not breathing normally.
- Check for signs of circulation.
- If no signs of circulation are present, start chest compressions.

✔ **Airway and Breathing:** Open the victim's airway by using the head tilt–chin lift technique, and then look, listen, and feel for breathing (use the jaw-thrust technique if trauma is present).

- Place your ear next to the victim's mouth and nose and look at the chest: **Look** for the chest to rise.
- **Listen** for breathing.
- **Feel** for air movement on your cheek.
- If the victim is not breathing, **provide 2 slow rescue breaths (about 2 seconds per breath).**
- Be sure the chest rises with each breath. If the chest does not rise, reopen the airway and reattempt rescue breaths.

✔ Check for **signs of circulation** (normal breathing, coughing, or movement in response to the 2 rescue breaths); if there are none, begin **chest compressions** at a rate of approximately 100 compressions per minute.

✔ During 1- and 2-rescuer CPR the ratio of compressions to rescue breaths is 15 to 2.

✔ After providing CPR for approximately 1 minute, recheck for signs of circulation.

✔ Place a victim who is unresponsive but breathing with signs of circulation in the recovery position.

✔ Perform the Heimlich maneuver (abdominal thrusts) for responsive victims with signs of severe or complete foreign-body airway obstruction. Place your fist just above the navel and well below the breastbone. If the victim becomes unresponsive, phone 911 and begin CPR (but look in the airway for a foreign object when you open the airway — remove any object you see).

Review Questions

1. **A coworker suddenly collapses. You gently shake him and shout, "Are you OK?" but he does not respond. You are alone so you shout for help. What do you do if no one responds to your shout?**

   a. phone 911 or other emergency response number (and get the AED if available), return to the victim and check for signs of circulation, open the airway, and give 2 breaths if the victim is not breathing

   b. open the airway, give 2 breaths if the victim is not breathing, check for signs of circulation, and phone 911 (and get the AED if available)

   c. phone 911 (and get the AED if available), return to the victim and open the airway, give 2 breaths if the victim is not breathing, and check for signs of circulation

   d. give 2 breaths if the victim is not breathing, check for signs of circulation, phone 911 (and get the AED if available), return to the victim and begin chest compressions

2. **You hear a coworker cry out in the next room. You enter the room and find him collapsed on the floor. What should your first action be?**

   a. check for breathing
   b. check for signs of circulation
   c. check for response
   d. open the airway

3. You are alone when you find your 68-year-old aunt lying unresponsive on the floor. You phone 911. There is no AED available in your home. You return and perform a head tilt–chin lift and look, listen, and feel for breathing. She is not breathing. What do you do next?

   a. give 2 rapid breaths
   b. give 2 slow breaths
   c. begin chest compressions
   d. place your aunt in the recovery position

4. A coworker at the table next to you complains of chest discomfort, turns pale, and collapses, falling to the floor. You determine that she is unresponsive and have someone phone 911 or other emergency response number (no AED is available). You perform a head tilt–chin lift and look, listen, and feel for breathing. The coworker is not breathing, so you provide 2 rescue breaths. The chest rises with each breath. You then check for signs of circulation. Which of the following are the signs of circulation you should look for?

   a. response to the rescue breaths (normal breathing, coughing, or movement)
   b. slow, gasping, irregular breaths
   c. blue, cool skin
   d. universal choking sign

5. The coworker described in question 4 has no signs of circulation. You begin chest compressions and ventilations. What is the correct ratio of compressions (pumping) to ventilations (blowing) that you should perform?

   a. 15 compressions to 2 breaths
   b. 10 compressions to 2 breaths
   c. 5 compressions to 2 breaths
   d. 5 compressions to 1 breath

6. You are playing cards with your neighbors when the wife collapses on the floor in the kitchen. You determine that she is unresponsive and ask her husband to phone 911 (no AED is available). You perform a head tilt–chin lift and then look, listen, and feel for breathing. You detect no breathing, so you deliver 2 rescue breaths. What do you look for to determine whether your rescue breaths are effective?

   a. a change in the color of the victim's skin
   b. blueness of the lips
   c. rising of the chest during rescue breathing
   d. a snoring noise during exhalation

7. While you are eating in a cafeteria you see an elderly man suddenly clutch his throat. He cannot cough, and he shakes his head "no" when you ask if he can speak. What should you do immediately?

   a. perform head tilt–chin lift
   b. give several back blows
   c. give abdominal thrusts
   d. phone 911 or other emergency response number

How did you do?

1, c; 2, c; 3, b; 4, a; 5, a; 6, c; 7, c.

Module 1

Chapter ③ *The Human Dimension of CPR*

The Human Dimension of CPR

Case Scenario

The day after you performed unsuccessful CPR on the beach for a father who had a heart attack, you awaken from a night of restless sleep. You feel fatigued, irritable, and confused. You keep replaying the scene of the resuscitation in your mind, wondering if you did everything correctly. You find that you are unable to stop thinking about the event. You call your family physician, and she invites you to her office to participate in what she calls a "critical incident stress debriefing." In this session you discuss your fears and feelings of guilt. By talking about the event, you come to realize that you are experiencing a common reaction to stress and that many people who receive CPR do not survive. You leave the session with a new perspective, taking comfort in knowing you took action and did your best.

How did the critical incident stress debriefing help you cope with this situation?

Learning Objectives

After reading this chapter, you should be able to

1. Explain how often CPR restores normal heartbeat and breathing in the out-of-hospital setting

2. Give 2 different definitions of "success" in resuscitation by a lay rescuer

3. State the importance of debriefing after a resuscitation attempt

4. Explain the role of the debriefing facilitator

5. Know how to contact an appropriate support person after a resuscitation attempt

The Human Dimension of CPR: How Often Will CPR Succeed?

Since 1973 more than 40 million people have learned CPR. Many public health experts consider CPR training to be the most successful public health initiative of modern times. Millions of people have been willing to prepare themselves to take action to save the life of a fellow human being. Unfortunately your best efforts will often be unsuccessful. CPR attempts at home or in public help restart the heart and restore breathing only about 50% of the time even in communities with the highest survival rates. Research tells us that training lay rescuers in citizen CPR courses will dramatically increase the number of survivors of cardiac arrest. Still the exact degree of success that can be achieved is unknown.

Even when their heart restarts, only about half of the victims of cardiac arrest due to VF who are admitted to the Emergency Department and the hospital survive and go home. This means that most of the time your CPR attempts will be unsuccessful. We think it is important to discuss the emotional reactions you and witnesses may have after a resuscitation attempt, especially when your efforts appear to have made no difference.

Take Pride in Your Skills as a Heartsaver Rescuer

You should be proud that you are learning CPR. We hope that you never have to use these skills. But emergencies happen. Now you can be confident that you will be better prepared to do the right thing for your family and loved ones, your coworkers, your neighbors, and even strangers.

Of course these emergencies can have negative outcomes. You and the emergency personnel who arrive to take over care may not restore the victim's life. Some people have a cardiac arrest simply because they have reached the end of a well-lived life. Your success will not be measured by whether a victim of cardiac arrest lives or dies. Your success will be measured by the fact that you tried. Simply by taking action, making an effort, and just trying to help you will be judged a success.

Stress Reactions of Rescuers and Witnesses After Resuscitation Attempts

A cardiac arrest is a dramatic and emotional event, especially if the victim is a friend or loved one. The emergency may involve disagreeable physical details, such as bleeding, vomiting, or poor hygiene. Any emergency can be an emotional burden, especially if the rescuer is closely involved with the victim. The emergency can produce strong emotional reactions in bystanders, lay rescuers, and EMS professionals. Failed attempts at resuscitation can be extremely stressful for rescuers. It will be even more stressful for you if you provide CPR for a family member, friend, or coworker. This stress can result in a variety of emotional reactions and physical symptoms that may last long after the original emergency. These reactions are common and normal.

It is **common** for a person to experience emotional aftershocks when he or she has experienced an unpleasant event. Usually such stress reactions occur immediately or within the first few hours after the event. Sometimes the emotional response occurs later.

Psychologists working with professional emergency personnel have learned that rescuers experience grief, anxiety, anger, and sometimes guilt. Typical physical reactions include difficulty sleeping, fatigue, irritability, changes in eating habits, and confusion. Many people say they are unable to stop thinking about the event.

Remember that these reactions are **common** and **normal.** They do not mean that you are "disturbed" or "weak." Strong reactions simply indicate that this particular event had a powerful impact on you. With the understanding and support of loved ones the stress reactions usually pass quickly.

Techniques to Prevent and Reduce Stress in Rescuers, Families, and Witnesses

Psychologists have learned that the most successful way to reduce stress after rescue efforts is very simple: **_Talk about it._** Sit down with other people who witnessed the event and talk it over. EMS personnel are encouraged to offer emotional support to lay rescuers and bystanders after both successful and unsuccessful resuscitation attempts. More formal discussions should include not only the lay rescuers but also the professional responders.

In these discussions you will be encouraged to describe what happened. Do not be afraid of "reliving" the event. Although such a fear is natural, talking about the event is a healthy way to deal with and overcome your fear. Describe the thoughts and feelings you experienced during the rescue effort. Describe how you feel now. Be patient with yourself. Understand that most reactions will diminish within a few days. Sharing your thoughts and feelings with your coworkers, fellow rescuers, EMS personnel, friends, or clergy can prevent or reduce stress reactions and help with your recovery.

In some locations (for example, the homes of high-risk patients or in the workplace), leaders of PAD programs may establish plans for more formal discussions or debriefings after resuscitation attempts. Such sessions have been called

critical incident stress debriefings, or critical event debriefings.

Teams of persons with special training are available to organize and conduct these CISDs. Such persons are usually associated with EMS services, employee assistance programs, community mental health centers, or public school systems. Other sources of psychological and emotional support can be local clergy, police chaplains, fire service chaplains, or hospital and Emergency Department social workers.

Critical event debriefings are a confidential group process. The facilitator leads and encourages persons involved in a stressful situation to express their thoughts and feelings about the event. You do not have to talk during the briefing, but if you do, what you say may help and reassure others. Rescuers and witnesses of an event can discuss shared feelings they experienced during and after a resuscitation attempt. These may be feelings of guilt, anxiety, or failure, especially if the outcome of the resuscitation attempt was negative. Ideally the rescuers who were most involved in the resuscitation should be present at the debriefing. In some PAD programs, EMS personnel visit lay rescuers who were involved in the resuscitative effort.

Psychological Barriers to Action

This course is preparing you to respond appropriately to a future emergency. Most laypersons have never been close to a victim of cardiac arrest and have seen CPR performed only on television or in the movies. Reality is quite different. While participating in the Heartsaver CPR Course or while reading this manual, you may have had some troubling thoughts.

Here are some common concerns lay rescuers express about responding to sudden cardiac emergencies. *Will I really have what it takes to respond to a true emergency?* Any emergency involving a friend, family member, or loved one

will produce strong emotional reactions. Parents, for example, sometimes feel paralyzed during the first few moments of an emergency involving their child. *Will I be able to take action?* and *Will I remember the steps of CPR and defibrillation?* These are common concerns.

What about the unpleasant and disagreeable aspects of doing CPR? Would you be able to perform mouth-to-mouth rescue breathing on a stranger? What if the victim is bleeding from facial injuries that occurred when he or she collapsed? What if a victim vomits during CPR? Would this pose a risk of disease for a rescuer without a CPR barrier device?

Often friends, relatives, or coworkers will be with you at the scene of an emergency. If you respond and take action, these people will often be willing to help, but they may look to you for instruction.
It may be difficult to act decisively at such an unexpected and challenging time.

These psychological barriers may hinder a quick emergency response, especially by ordinary citizens who seldom face such an event. There are no easy solutions to help someone overcome these barriers. Think through how you would plan to respond if confronted with an emergency. Mental practice, even without hands-on practice, is a good technique for improving future performance.

The AHA Emergency Cardiovascular Care Committee encourages you to attend routine skills review and practice sessions at least every 6 months. The required renewal interval for this course is **every 2 years.** Review and practice sessions and renewal courses will strengthen your skills, build your confidence, and increase the probability of a smooth and effective resuscitative effort. Most Heartsaver CPR programs in the workplace will provide review sessions to help you remain focused on the task at hand: performing the links in the Chain of Survival (phoning 911 or other emergency response number and providing CPR) to save a life.

Legal Aspects of CPR

The AHA has supported community CPR training for more than 3 decades. Lay rescuers have helped save thousands of lives by providing CPR.

Lay responders can perform emergency CPR without fear of legal action. Chest compressions and rescue breathing require direct physical contact between rescuer and victim, 2 people who may be strangers. Too often the victim of cardiac arrest dies. In the United States people may take legal action when they perceive damage or think that one person has harmed another even if the harm was unintentional. Despite this litigious environment, CPR remains widely used and remarkably free of legal issues and lawsuits. Although attorneys have included rescuers who performed CPR in lawsuits, no "Good Samaritan" has ever been found guilty of doing harm while performing CPR.

All 50 states have Good Samaritan laws that grant immunity to anyone who attempts CPR in an honest, "good faith" effort to save a life. A lay rescuer or lay responder is considered a Good Samaritan if

- The rescuer is genuinely trying to help
- The help is reasonable (the rescuer cannot engage in gross misconduct)
- The rescue effort is voluntary (the rescuer is not paid for the resuscitative effort)

Under most Good Samaritan laws, laypersons are protected if they perform CPR even if they have had no formal training.

Summary

Be proud of your initiative to take a course in CPR. Be proud of your new skills as a lay rescuer who can perform CPR to save a life.

Despite all the excitement about CPR and public access defibrillation, there are limitations to what you can do. Your efforts will not always succeed. What is important is to take action and try to help another human being. Some people must overcome psychological barriers to action if asked to respond to a dramatic emergency such as cardiac arrest. Taking the Heartsaver CPR Course will reduce many of these barriers. Feel free to express your concerns openly during the course and small-group sessions.

All Heartsaver lay responders are encouraged to be aware of the mental and emotional challenge of rescue efforts. You will have support if you ever participate in a resuscitation attempt. You may not know for several days whether the victim lives or dies. If the person you tried to resuscitate does not live, take comfort in knowing that in taking action you did your best.

Learning Checklist

✔ CPR attempts are often unsuccessful. Your efforts will not always succeed in restoring life.

✔ The best way to reduce stress after a rescue effort is to talk about it.

✔ Formal discussions or debriefings after resuscitations are called critical incident stress debriefings.

✔ Some people must overcome psychological barriers to action if asked to respond to a cardiac arrest.

✔ There has never been a lawsuit in which a lay rescuer was found guilty of doing harm in attempting CPR on a victim of cardiac arrest.

✔ Your success will be measured by the fact that you tried.

Review Questions

1. **A friend who helped you perform CPR 2 days ago says she is experiencing fatigue, irritability, difficulty sleeping, guilt, loss of appetite, shortness of breath, anxiety, and depression. What is the most likely cause of these symptoms?**

   a. heart attack

   b. a virus that she caught while performing CPR

   c. stress response

   d. heart failure

2. **Your friend who is experiencing the symptoms described in question 1 asks what she should do to address this problem. You suggest that she attend a group meeting led by a physician, social worker, or other professional in which she can express her feelings. What is the term for this type of meeting?**

   a. critical incident stress debriefing

   b. analysis

   c. biofeedback

   d. psychological ventilation

3. **An emergency physician approaches you after an unsuccessful resuscitation attempt to ask how he and his associates can help to reduce your stress after the event. What role might you suggest for the physician that would be helpful to you and other rescuers after a resuscitation attempt?**

   a. facilitator of a debriefing process

   b. observer of a debriefing process

   c. passive participant

   d. no particular role

How did you do?

1, c; **2**, a; **3**, a.

Appendixes
Adult CPR

Heartsaver CPR Course for Adults

Adult 1-Rescuer CPR Performance Criteria

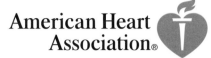

American Heart Association®

Fighting Heart Disease and Stroke

Student Name_____   Date _____

Performance Guidelines	Performed
1. Establish that the victim is unresponsive. Phone 911 (or other emergency response number).	
2. Open airway (head tilt–chin lift or, if trauma is suspected, jaw thrust). Check for normal breathing (look, listen, and feel).*	
3. If normal breathing is absent, give 2 slow breaths (2 seconds per breath), ensure adequate chest rise, and allow for exhalation between breaths.	
4. Check for signs of circulation (normal breathing, coughing, or movement in response to the 2 rescue breaths). If signs of circulation are present but there is no normal breathing, provide rescue breathing (1 breath every 5 seconds, about 10 to 12 breaths per minute).	
5. If no signs of circulation are present, begin cycles of 15 chest compressions (about 100 compressions per minute) followed by 2 slow breaths.*	
6. After 4 cycles of compressions and breaths (15:2, about 1 minute), recheck for signs of circulation.* If no signs of circulation are present, continue 15:2 cycles, beginning with chest compressions. If signs of circulation return but breathing does not, continue rescue breathing (1 breath every 5 seconds, or about 10 to 12 breaths per minute).	

*If the victim is breathing or resumes normal breathing and no trauma is suspected, place in the recovery position.

Comments _____

_____

_____

Instructor _____

Circle one: Complete   Needs more practice

Heartsaver CPR Course for Adults

Adult 2-Rescuer CPR
Performance Criteria

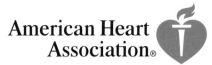

American Heart
Association®

Fighting Heart Disease and Stroke

Student Name_____ Date _____

Performance Guidelines	Performed
1. Establish that the victim is unresponsive. One rescuer should first phone 911 (or other emergency response number).	
Rescuer 1	
2. Open the airway (head tilt–chin lift or, if trauma is suspected, jaw thrust). Check for normal breathing (look, listen, and feel).*	
3. If normal breathing is absent, give 2 slow breaths (2 seconds per breath), ensure adequate chest rise, and allow for exhalation between breaths.	
4. Check for signs of circulation (normal breathing, coughing, or movement in response to the 2 rescue breaths). If signs of circulation are present but there is no normal breathing, provide rescue breathing (1 breath every 5 seconds, about 10 to 12 breaths per minute).	
Rescuer 2	
5. If no signs of circulation are present, begin cycles of 15 chest compressions (rate of about 100 compressions per minute) followed by 2 slow breaths by Rescuer 1.*	
6. After 4 cycles of compressions and breaths (15:2, about 1 minute), rescuer 1 provides 2 breaths and rechecks for signs of circulation.* If no signs of circulation are present, continue 15:2 cycles of compressions and ventilations, beginning with chest compressions, until more skilled rescuers (with an AED) arrive.	

*If the victim is breathing or resumes effective breathing and no trauma is suspected, place in the recovery position.

Comments _____

_____

Instructor _____

Circle one: Complete   Needs more practice

Adult Foreign-Body Airway Obstruction in Responsive Victim
(and Responsive Victim Who Becomes Unresponsive)
Performance Criteria

American Heart Association®

Fighting Heart Disease and Stroke

Student Name _____   Date _____

Performance Guidelines	Performed
1. Ask "Are you choking?" If yes, ask "Can you speak?" If no, tell the victim you are going to help.	
2. Give abdominal thrusts (chest thrusts for victim who is pregnant or obese). Avoid pressing on the bottom of the breastbone (xiphoid).	
3. Repeat thrusts until foreign body is expelled (obstruction relieved) or victim becomes unresponsive.	
Adult Foreign-Body Airway Obstruction — Victim Becomes Unresponsive The following is for clarification only. It is not to be emphasized or evaluated in the lay rescuer course.	
4. Phone 911 or other emergency response number (or send someone to do it). Return to the victim.	
5. Attempt CPR (each time you open the airway, look for a foreign object in the mouth; if you see it, remove it).	

Comments _____

_____

_____

_____

_____

_____

Instructor _____

Circle one: Complete   Needs more practice

Appendix B

Special Resuscitation Situations

The direction to call 911 or other emergency response number first for adult victims is based on the most likely causes of collapse in adults and the actions that are most likely to produce survival. In adults the most likely cause of witnessed arrest is cardiac arrest resulting from ventricular fibrillation, a lethal cardiac rhythm that causes the heart to quiver, preventing it from pumping blood. Although CPR will help, this condition will not resolve until defibrillation (shocking the heart with a defibrillator) is provided. The sooner defibrillation occurs, the better the victim's chance of survival. For this reason, the rescuer of an adult victim should phone 911 (or other emergency response number) first to get EMS personnel to the scene with a defibrillator as soon as possible.

Usually more than 1 person is present at the scene of an emergency. In such cases the trained rescuer should direct someone to phone 911 or other emergency response number (and get the AED if available) while the trained rescuer begins CPR. This allows the first 2 links of the Chain of Survival to be accomplished at the same time. Only in the case of a single rescuer does the sequence of phoning first and then beginning CPR become important.

Following are exceptions to the rule of "Phone First!" (phone 911 or other emergency response number before beginning CPR for adults). These exceptions apply only in situations in which only 1 rescuer is available. The most likely cause of collapse or arrest in the 3 cases described below is a blocked airway or lack of adequate breathing. In these 3 cases, if you are alone, you should **perform CPR first** for approximately 1 minute before phoning 911 (or other emergency

response number). This action will deliver oxygen to the vital organs and may restore circulation and breathing.

Submersion/Near-Drowning

Lack of oxygen is the most important problem caused by submersion or near-drowning. The longer the victim is without oxygen, the greater the chance of death or damage to the brain. For this reason, rescue breathing and chest compressions (if needed) should be started *as soon as the victim is pulled from the water.* When you rescue a near-drowning victim, provide rescue breathing and other steps of CPR for about 1 minute and then phone 911. Do not leave the victim to phone 911 first, because that would prolong the victim's time without oxygen and increase the chance of death or damage to the brain.

You must keep yourself safe when attempting to rescue a victim of near-drowning. Pull the victim to a secure place to begin CPR. If it is possible that the victim dived or fell into the water, assume that a head or neck injury is present and avoid bending the neck or turning the head. The victim may have a broken neck, so open the airway by using the jaw thrust (instead of head tilt–chin lift).

Respiratory and Cardiac Arrest Caused by Injury

Breathing and circulation may stop after a severe injury, such as one caused by a car crash. Some injured victims stop breathing but do not have a cardiac arrest. If you begin the steps of CPR immediately, you increase the victim's chance of survival. Do not delay CPR to phone 911. In injured victims damage to the jaw and facial bones may cause airway obstruction. If the victim suffers a head injury and becomes unresponsive, the tongue may block the airway. By opening the airway and providing rescue breathing, you may save the victim's life. Open the airway with *jaw thrust* (instead of head tilt–chin lift) because the neck may be injured. If the victim has no signs of circulation, perform chest compressions. Perform CPR for about 1 minute, then leave the victim to phone 911.

The victim must be on a firm, flat surface if chest compressions are required. If it is necessary to move the victim to the ground or to roll the victim onto his or her back, be careful to move the head, neck, and body as one unit. Prevent bending or twisting of the neck and back.

Drug Overdose

It may be hard to determine whether a victim has taken an overdose of drugs. If you are certain that an overdose was the cause of the collapse, provide CPR for about 1 minute and then leave the victim to phone 911 and get the AED if one is available. The most common problem caused by an overdose is breathing difficulty or respiratory arrest. These victims need immediate rescue breathing. Chest compressions are usually not needed, but be prepared to provide them if necessary.

Summary

Remember, if you are alone with an adult who is unresponsive, in general you should phone 911 (or other emergency response number) first. In a small number of situations you should perform CPR (this may include rescue breathing alone or breathing plus compressions) for approximately 1 minute and then phone 911 (or other emergency response number). This approach will increase the likelihood of survival. You should perform CPR for about 1 minute before leaving the victim to phone 911 if you suspect the victim's lack of response is caused by one of the following 3 conditions:

- Near-drowning/submersion
- Injury
- Drug overdose

Action Scenarios: Applying Your Knowledge of CPR

This appendix presents **study cases** to help you learn how to apply the skills of CPR. The following **cases** review different situations that you may face as a rescuer. Each case illustrates a common emergency that requires a unique action. For each case do the following:

- Cover the answer below the case with a piece of paper and then carefully review the case.

- Think about the single **best** answer to the question.
- Write your answer in the space provided.
- Review the correct answer and the rationale for the answer.
- If the answer and discussion are unclear, review the related section in this manual.
- If you have additional questions, ask your Heartsaver CPR Course instructor.

CASE 1: A Coworker With Chest Pain

Your 53-year-old coworker clutches his chest while at the elevator. He says he has "pressure-like" chest pain that has lasted for about 5 minutes. His skin is cool, pale, and sweaty, and he says he feels nauseated and dizzy. He tells you that this has never happened to him before today. What immediate actions do you take?

What is your answer?

_____

_____

Why? _____

_____

_____

Case 1 Answer: Your coworker is exhibiting the classic signs of a heart attack. Place him in a comfortable resting position and immediately phone 911 (or other emergency response number). It is important to phone 911 immediately for 2 reasons. First, the victim's risk of developing abnormal heart rhythms is highest during the first *hour* after the onset of symptoms. Second, the victim may be eligible for treatments such as clotbuster medications, which can decrease damage to the victim's heart and prevent cardiac arrest. These drugs must be given within the first few hours after the onset of symptoms. Be careful — victims of heart attack will often deny that they are having a problem and refuse to seek medical attention. In such circumstances make every attempt to convince the victim to seek help immediately.

CASE 2: Your Supervisor Has Difficulty Speaking and Moving

Your 62-year-old supervisor is chairing a lunch meeting when she suddenly seems confused. You notice a facial droop in the corner of her mouth, and she cannot move her left arm and leg. She is also slurring her words when she speaks. She tells you that she is fine and that you shouldn't worry. What actions should you take?

What is your answer?

_____

_____

Why?   _____

_____

_____

Case 2 Answer: Your supervisor is exhibiting the classic signs of a stroke. Immediately phone 911. It is important for you to phone 911 (or other emergency response number) immediately for several reasons. Most important, treatments such as clotbuster medications can decrease the risk and extent of brain damage. These treatments *must* be given within the *first few hours* after the onset of symptoms. EMS personnel can confirm that your supervisor has likely suffered a stroke, and they can notify the hospital Emergency Department that a patient with a possible stroke will be arriving soon. This will reduce delays at the hospital and increase the likelihood that your supervisor will arrive and be evaluated within the 3-hour window to receive clotbuster medications. Closely monitor the victim until emergency personnel arrive. Complications such as airway obstruction or respiratory arrest (the victim stops breathing) can develop, and the victim may need your help to maintain an open airway. You may also need to provide rescue breathing. Never allow a stroke victim to deny the emergency. Seek help immediately!

CASE 3: A Near-Drowning Victim

Your neighbor yells for help. When you arrive in her backyard, you see a 25-year-old man floating face down in the swimming pool. You and your neighbor pull the victim from the pool, and you note that he is unresponsive. You send your neighbor to phone 911 immediately. You open the victim's airway with a jaw thrust and check for breathing. You note that the victim is not breathing, and you give 2 slow breaths, then you check for signs of circulation. After the 2 rescue breaths the victim moves his arms and legs, but his breathing is inadequate. What actions should you take?

What is your answer?

_____

_____

Why?   _____

_____

_____

Case 3 Answer: You should continue to provide rescue breaths at a rate of 1 breath every 5 seconds (about 10 to 12 breaths per minute). Respiratory arrest (the victim stops breathing) with effective circulation is common in many emergencies, such as near-drowning, drug overdose, stroke, electrocution, and head injury. Victims who are in respiratory arrest but have other signs of circulation (normal breathing, coughing, movement) do not require chest compressions. Continue to provide rescue breathing and monitor the victim's signs of circulation until emergency personnel arrive. If the signs of circulation disappear, immediately start chest compressions with rescue breaths at a ratio of 15 compressions to 2 breaths. In cases of near-drowning you should also think about injury to the spine. If the victim was diving into shallow water, there is a risk of injury to the spinal column. If you think the victim may have a spinal injury, be careful to keep the spine in alignment when removing the victim from the water and use the jaw thrust (not the head tilt–chin lift) to open and maintain the victim's airway.

CASE 4: A Handyman Is Electrocuted

Local contractors are remodeling a wing of the company headquarters. You are at work, and you hear a call for help from the construction area. On arrival you find a 45-year-old man having a seizure. He is holding an electrical wire. The victim's coworker pulls the plug from the wall that leads to the wire in the victim's hand, and the seizure stops. As soon as you are sure the area is safe, you assess the victim and note that he is unresponsive. You have the coworker immediately phone 911 or other emergency response number (and get the AED if available) and you open the victim's airway and check for breathing. The victim is not breathing. After you provide 2 rescue breaths, you find that the victim has no signs of circulation. What actions should you take?

What is your answer?

_____

_____

Why? _____

_____

_____

Case 4 Answer: You should immediately start chest compressions and provide chest compressions and ventilations at a ratio of 15 compressions to 2 breaths. Tell the coworker to advise the 911 dispatcher that the victim is in cardiac arrest. Defibrillation is the key treatment for any adult victim of cardiac arrest and is almost always useful for victims of electrocution, who are likely to have VF. Recheck for signs of circulation after about 1 minute and every few minutes thereafter until emergency personnel arrive.

CASE 5: An Emergency at the Cafeteria

You are eating at the cafeteria when a 32-year-old friend sitting at the end of the table suddenly appears to be in distress. She is clutching her throat and struggling to breathe. You approach her and ask, "Are you choking?" She nods her head. You ask, "Can you speak?" She shakes her head back and forth, but you don't hear any sounds. What actions should you take?

What is your answer?

_____

_____

Why? _____

_____

_____

Case 5 Answer: Immediately position yourself behind the victim and place your fist just above the navel and well below the breastbone. Provide several abdominal thrusts until the foreign object is expelled or the victim becomes unresponsive. If the victim becomes unresponsive, have some-one phone 911 (or other emergency response number) immediately while you begin CPR (if you are alone, you phone 911 and then begin CPR). Every time you open the airway, open it widely and look for an object. If you see an object in the back of the throat, remove it. If you do not see an object, continue to provide compressions and ventilations.

CASE 6: A Coworker Is Not Breathing After Return of Circulation

Your 48-year-old coworker suddenly collapses at her desk. You note that she is unresponsive, so you direct another coworker to phone 911 immediately. You open the victim's airway and check for breathing. She is not breathing, so you provide 2 slow breaths. After the 2 breaths you note that she has no signs of circulation.

You immediately start chest compressions. After providing compressions and ventilations for 1 minute, you recheck for signs of circulation. The victim is moving her arms and legs but is not breathing. What actions should you take?

What is your answer?

_____

_____

Why?   _____

_____

_____

Case 6 Answer: You should continue to provide rescue breaths at a rate of 1 breath every 5 seconds. Respiratory arrest (the victim stops breathing) is common after return of circulation with successful CPR or defibrillation. When the brain is deprived of oxygen for even a short period of time, a recovery interval is needed to restore normal brain function, including responsiveness and breathing. Continue rescue breathing until emergency personnel arrive.

Glossary of Terms

Angina — A condition in which the heart muscle receives an insufficient supply of blood, causing temporary pain in the chest and often the left arm and shoulder. Angina usually occurs during physical activity or when a person is emotionally upset.

Artery — A blood vessel that carries blood away from the heart to the various parts of the body.

Automated External Defibrillator (AED) — A computerized medical device that identifies irregular ("shockable") heart rhythms, specifically ventricular tachycardia and ventricular fibrillation. If a shockable rhythm is detected, the AED charges to an appropriate shock dose and advises the operator to deliver an electric shock to the cardiac arrest victim in an attempt to allow a normal heart rhythm to resume. Lay rescuers can operate an AED for use in adults and children 8 years of age or older who are in cardiac arrest (no response, no normal breathing, no signs of circulation). The AED assesses the victim's cardiac rhythm to determine whether a rhythm that will respond to shocks is present. If such a rhythm is detected, the AED "advises" the operator to press the SHOCK button. See **Defibrillator.**

Barrier Devices — Plastic or silicon devices that allow a rescuer to provide rescue breathing without coming into direct contact with the victim's mouth or nose. The devices are placed over the victim's mouth and nose. There are 2 types of barrier devices: *face shields*, which are flexible and mold closely to the face, and *face masks*, which are rigid and increase the distance between the victim and the rescuer.

Blood Pressure — The force of pressure exerted by the heart in pumping blood; the pressure of blood in the arteries.

Cardiac Arrest — A condition in which the heart suddenly stops pumping blood. Sudden cardiac arrest in adults is most often caused by an abnormal heart rhythm, usually ventricular fibrillation (VF). The victim in cardiac arrest shows no response to stimuli, no normal breathing, and no signs of circulation (no normal breathing, coughing, or movement in response to 2 rescue breaths).

Cardiopulmonary Resuscitation (CPR) — A series of steps that include opening the airway, assessing breathing, providing rescue breathing, assessing signs of circulation, and providing chest compressions. These actions keep oxygen-rich blood flowing to the brain and heart until defibrillation and advanced life support can be provided.

Cardiovascular — Pertaining to the heart and blood vessels, including the major blood vessels that supply blood to the brain.

Circulatory System — The heart and blood vessels (arteries, veins, and capillaries).

Coronary Arteries — Blood vessels arising from the aorta and circling the surface of the heart to conduct blood to the heart muscle.

Coronary Care Unit (CCU) — An in-hospital specialized facility or emergency mobile unit equipped with monitoring devices, staffed with trained personnel, and designed to treat patients who have had a heart attack or other serious heart conditions.

Coronary Occlusion — An obstruction or narrowing of a coronary artery that hinders or completely blocks blood flow to part of the heart muscle. See **Heart Attack.**

Coronary Thrombosis — Formation of a clot in an artery that conducts blood to the heart muscle. Also called *coronary occlusion.*

Defibrillation — Successful treatment of ventricular fibrillation using electric shocks delivered by a defibrillator.

Defibrillator — A medical device that delivers an electric current to the heart to treat ventricular fibrillation. The current is delivered through either adhesive electrode pads that are attached to the chest or through handheld metal paddles. Defibrillators can be either automated or manual. Manual defibrillators are operated by healthcare providers, but automated external defibrillators (AEDs) can be operated by healthcare providers or lay rescuers in communities with public access defibrillation programs. See **Automated External Defibrillator.**

Endotracheal Tube or Tracheal Tube — A plastic tube inserted from the mouth into the windpipe of a victim who is not breathing effectively (may be called a "breathing tube"). Advanced healthcare personnel (ie, doctors, nurses, and paramedics) may insert endotracheal or tracheal tubes.

Heart Attack — A nonspecific term usually referring to the death of heart muscle caused by complete blockage of a diseased coronary artery by a blood clot. *Myocardial infarction* is a more specific term for what is usually meant by *heart attack.*

High Blood Pressure (Hypertension) — Persistent elevation of blood pressure above the normal range.

Myocardial Infarction — See **Heart Attack.**

Myocardium — Heart muscle.

Nitroglycerin — A drug that causes dilation of blood vessels, including blood vessels supplying the heart. This drug is often used to treat angina.

Occluded Artery — An artery in which blood flow is impaired by a blockage.

Public Access Defibrillation (PAD) — A public health initiative developed by the American Heart Association. PAD encourages the development of programs that install automated external defibrillators (AEDs) throughout the community and train rescuers to use them. PAD programs require physician supervision and contact with the local emergency medical services (EMS) system. In communities with a PAD program, AEDs can be used by a large number of rescuers, including firefighters, police officers, security guards, and even family members of high-risk patients. Quick, accurate use of an AED can substantially shorten the time to defibrillation and improve the chance of survival of victims of out-of-hospital cardiac arrest.

Pulmonary — Pertaining to the lungs.

Respiratory Arrest — A condition in which a victim is not breathing at all or is breathing so slowly, shallowly, or irregularly that adequate oxygenation of the blood cannot occur. To distinguish it from *cardiac arrest,* this term is reserved for victims who are not breathing effectively but who still have signs of circulation.

Stroke — A sudden onset of weakness or paralysis on one side of the body (such as one arm or leg) caused by an insufficient supply of blood to part of the brain. A stroke can affect balance, coordination, speech, and vision. Older terms for stroke are *apoplexy, cerebrovascular accident,* and *cerebral vascular accident.*

Vascular — Pertaining to the blood vessels.

Vein — Any one of a series of vessels of the cardiovascular system that carry blood from various parts of the body back to the heart.

Ventricular Fibrillation (VF) — A chaotic, uncoordinated quivering of the cardiac muscle that prevents effective contraction of the heart. VF causes cardiac arrest; biological death follows within minutes if VF is not treated. Defibrillation is the treatment needed for VF. A defibrillator is used to deliver a strong electric shock to the heart. When this shock is successful, the heart is "stunned," and a normal rhythm resumes (defibrillation has occurred).

Appendix E

Frequently Asked Questions About CPR

1. Can rescuers catch AIDS, hepatitis, or other diseases during CPR?

It is extremely unlikely that a rescuer will become infected with human immunodeficiency virus (HIV), the virus that causes AIDS, or any of the hepatitis viruses as a result of performing mouth-to-mouth breathing or touching the victim. CPR (including mouth-to-mouth breathing) has been performed for more than 35 years, and there has never been a documented case of transmission of HIV or any hepatitis virus from a victim to a rescuer. You can use a face mask or a face shield as a barrier device, but such a device is not necessary to perform CPR. The face shield prevents contact with the victim's mouth and face. The mask contains a 1-way valve to help block the transmission of viruses and bacteria between the victim and rescuer.

It is important for rescuers to know that most respiratory and cardiac arrests (70% to 80%) occur in the home, where the rescuer usually knows the victim and knows about the victim's health conditions. A primary reason to learn CPR is for the benefit of your family and friends. Barrier devices should be available for all rescuers who provide CPR in the workplace.

2. What are some possible hazards of CPR?

CPR can cause injuries. To reduce the risk of potential complications of CPR, follow performance guidelines at all times. Frequent practice with a manikin helps improve future performance.

Possible problems in performing CPR that may contribute to complications include the following:

- Incorrect positioning of the hands for chest compressions may lead to rib fractures, fractures of the end of the breastbone (xiphoid), and bruising or bleeding of the liver, lung, or spleen.

- Bouncing chest compressions may cause the rescuer's hands to move off the center of the sternum (breastbone) so that other structures (ribs, lung, liver) are compressed and possibly injured.
- Compressing the chest too deeply may cause internal injury.
- Not compressing the sternum deeply enough may provide insufficient blood flow to the brain and other vital organs.
- Providing a volume of breath that is too great, breathing too rapidly, or not opening the airway completely may cause you to blow large amounts of air into the stomach, causing the stomach to fill with air (gastric inflation). Gastric inflation increases the chances that the victim will vomit and may decrease the effectiveness of ventilations.

3. How do I open the airway of a victim who may have a neck injury, such as a victim of a car crash?

Use a *jaw thrust* to open the airway of a victim suspected of having a neck injury.

4. What should I do if the victim vomits?

If the victim vomits and no injury to the head or neck is suspected, turn the victim's head and body to the side so that the victim will not choke on the vomited material. If you suspect a head or neck injury, turn the head, neck, and entire body to the side as a unit ("log roll" the victim) without flexing or turning the neck. Then clear the airway by sweeping the mouth. A cloth (for example, a corner of clothing or handkerchief) wrapped around your fingers can be used to sweep the mouth. Then reposition the victim and continue CPR. If injury to the head or neck is suspected, you *must* turn the head, neck, and body as one unit.

5. How will I know if signs of circulation and breathing return?

The return of signs of circulation, with or without breathing, may be dramatic or subtle. The victim may take a big gasp of air, begin moving, cough, or even start to become responsive. If normal breathing also returns, keep the airway open and regularly check for signs of circulation and breathing. Place the victim in the recovery position to maintain an open airway. If an adult victim is not breathing normally (for example, making only occasional attempts at gasping), continue to perform rescue breathing at a rate of about 10 to 12 breaths per minute (once every 5 seconds).

6. What should I do about a "neck breather" who needs CPR?

"Neck breathers" are persons who have a permanent opening (stoma) that connects the airway or windpipe (trachea) directly to the skin of the neck. The opening is at the base of the front of the neck. To tell whether the victim's breathing has returned, place your ear over the opening in the neck. If rescue breathing is required, perform mouth-to-stoma rescue breathing (put your mouth over the opening in the neck to provide rescue breaths). For more information, contact the International Association of Laryngectomees, ℅ American Cancer Society, 1599 Clifton Rd NE, Atlanta, GA 30329.

7. If a victim is lying on a bed, should I move him to the floor so that a hard surface is under his back?

Victims who need CPR should be moved to a firm level surface if at all possible, so you should move the victim to the floor. Make sure that the victim's head and neck are well supported. If you are alone and cannot move the victim, leave the victim on the bed and try to find something flat and firm (such as an ironing board or other board) to slide under the victim's back to provide a firm surface. If you cannot immediately locate something to place under the victim and you absolutely cannot move him, begin CPR with the victim on the bed (do not delay). Try to compress the chest with enough force that the breastbone moves inward about 1½ to 2 inches. You won't be able to create blood flow if you simply push the victim into the bed.

8. What should I do if the victim is wearing dentures?

Leave the dentures in place if possible. This will help you make an airtight seal around the victim's mouth. Remove the dentures only if they are so loose or ill-fitting that they get in your way or obstruct the victim's airway.

9. What should I do to prevent air from filling the stomach (gastric inflation)?

Inflation of the stomach (air getting into the stomach) is most likely to occur if you blow too hard or too fast during rescue breathing or if the airway is partially obstructed. Control the force and speed of rescue breaths. Breathe slowly into the victim, taking 2 seconds to deliver each breath, and blow in only enough air to make the chest rise.

10. What if the victim of complete airway obstruction is pregnant or obese?

Treat the pregnant or obese victim of choking the same way as any other victim unless it is impossible to perform safe or effective abdominal thrusts because the pregnancy is advanced or the obesity is extreme. In these cases perform chest thrusts instead of abdominal thrusts.

11. How will I know when to perform abdominal thrusts on a choking victim?

If the victim is moving air (in other words, the foreign body is *not* completely obstructing the airway), the victim will cough forcefully, although you may hear wheezing between coughs. As long as good air exchange continues, encourage the victim to keep coughing and breathing. At this point do not interfere with the victim's attempts to expel the foreign body. A victim with *severe or complete* airway obstruction will be unable to speak, breathe, or cough forcefully. The victim also may clutch his or her neck (the universal sign of choking). If the victim cannot speak, you must try to relieve the obstruction with abdominal thrusts (the Heimlich maneuver).

12. *How often should I review or renew my skills in CPR?*

The AHA Emergency Cardiovascular Care Committee recommends retraining at least every 2 years to renew your CPR skills. The committee encourages you to practice your CPR skills frequently within this time period.

Appendix F

Self-Test Questions

Please take the following self-test. If you are unsure of an answer, review the material on the pages listed below the item.

1. **A coworker suddenly staggers and collapses in front of you. What do you do next?**

   a. phone 911 or other emergency response number

   b. perform a head tilt–chin lift and look, listen, and feel for breathing

   c. check to see if the coworker is responsive

   d. check for signs of circulation

   Answer is **c**; see page 24.

2. **You are alone when you discover an employee of the shopping mall collapsed in an aisle with no signs of a fall or injury. You gently shake him and shout, "Are you OK?" He doesn't respond, so you phone 911 (or other emergency response number). What do you do next?**

   a. give 2 rescue breaths

   b. perform a head tilt–chin lift and look, listen, and feel for breathing

   c. establish that the victim is unresponsive

   d. check for signs of circulation

   Answer is **b**; see page 25.

3. **You have opened the employee's airway, confirmed that he is not breathing, and given 2 slow rescue breaths. What do you do next?**

   a. get an AED

   b. perform a head tilt–chin lift and look, listen, and feel for breathing

   c. perform chest compressions

   d. check for signs of circulation

   Answer is **d**; see page 26.

4. **You have performed about 1 minute of CPR on an employee in the mall with a compression ("pumping") to breathing ("blowing") ratio of 15:2. You know that about 1 minute has elapsed because you can see a clock on the wall. What do you do next?**

   a. place the victim in the recovery position

   b. check for signs of circulation

   c. begin chest compressions

   d. give 2 rescue breaths

   Answer is **b**; see page 26.

5. **After several minutes of CPR, the employee shows signs of circulation by moving his arms and legs. What do you do next?**

   a. perform a head tilt–chin lift and look, listen, and feel for breathing

   b. place the victim in the recovery position

   c. begin chest compressions

   d. give 2 rescue breaths

   Answer is **a**; see pages 24-25.

6. **The employee continues to show signs of circulation but is not breathing. What do you do next?**

   a. perform rescue breathing with a compression ("pumping") to breathing ("blowing") ratio of 15:2

   b. perform rescue breathing with a compression ("pumping") to breathing ("blowing") ratio of 5:1

   c. perform rescue breathing at a rate of 1 breath every 5 seconds (about 10 to 12 per minute)

   d. place the victim in the recovery position to maintain an open airway

   Answer is **c**; see page 26.

7. **During dinner at the cafeteria your 22-year-old friend suddenly stops talking, clutches her neck, and appears to be in distress. What do you do next?**

   a. phone 911 or other emergency response number
   b. perform a head tilt–chin lift and look, listen, and feel for breathing
   c. shake her and see if she responds
   d. ask her, "Are you choking?" If she nods yes, ask, "Can you speak?"

   Answer is **d**; see page 15.

8. **Your friend responds by beginning to cough forcefully with very noisy breath sounds and says, "Went down the wrong way." What should you do next?**

   a. phone 911 or other emergency response number and be sure she is evaluated by a doctor
   b. perform a head tilt–chin lift to open the airway
   c. perform abdominal thrusts
   d. do not interfere but monitor the situation

   Answer is **d**; see page 15.

9. **You are alone with a 52-year-old man at the bus stop who becomes pale and sweaty and complains of terrible "pressure" in his chest. No other bystanders are present. What do you do next?**

   a. tell the man to sit on the bench and remain there while you call 911 from a nearby pay telephone
   b. stay with the man and be prepared to perform CPR
   c. do not interfere but monitor the situation
   d. place the man in the recovery position

   Answer is **a**; see pages 10-11.

10. **Your 72-year-old neighbor calls for help. When you go to her apartment, you note that she has a facial droop, arm weakness, and difficulty speaking. What do you do next?**

    a. drive her to the hospital immediately
    b. contact her doctor's answering service
    c. contact her next of kin
    d. phone 911

    Answer is **d**; see pages 13-14.

Module 2

Infant and Child CPR and Prevention of Injuries and Arrest

Module 2

Chapter ❶ Early Action Saves Lives
The Chain of Survival and Recognition of Life-Threatening Emergencies in Infants and Children

1

Early Action Saves Lives
The Chain of Survival and
Recognition of Life-Threatening
Emergencies in Infants and Children

Case Scenario

You are walking on a beach, and you notice a family enjoying a picnic near the water. You see an elderly man, a middle-aged man, a young child, and an infant sitting on a blanket eating lunch. As you walk by the family, you overhear some of the conversation, allowing you to identify a grandfather, a father, a 3-year-old son, and a 10-month-old son. You speak briefly to the family and then continue walking for several minutes. Suddenly you hear someone shout from the direction you have come: "Help! I think he needs CPR! I don't know what to do! Somebody help me!"

As you run toward the shout, you realize you are running toward the family picnic. You wonder who needs CPR. Is it the grandfather, the father, the child, or the infant?

You arrive at the site of the family picnic and see a man standing waist high in the water holding a limp child. You rush toward the man as he carries the child out of the water and lays him on the sand. You recognize the father and the 3-year-old son you spoke with a few moments ago. The child is limp and does not respond to voice or touch. His lips are blue. The man says, "He just went under. I got to him as fast as I could, but I had trouble finding him under the water. I don't know what to do. Can you help me?"

How would you assess the child's condition and what should be your first action if the child is not responsive? Does this scenario represent a typical cause of cardiopulmonary arrest in a child? Could it have been prevented? How?

What should you do? Describe your actions and how they become the critical links in the AHA pediatric Chain of Survival.

Learning Objectives

After reading this chapter you should be able to

1. Name the links in the AHA pediatric Chain of Survival and discuss the role you play in the chain.
2. List the warning signs of these 3 major emergencies in infants and children:
   a. Breathing problems requiring emergency care
   b. Cardiac arrest
   c. Foreign-body airway obstruction (choking)
3. Describe how and when to activate the EMS system.

AHA Pediatric Chain of Survival

In the United States the leading cause of death in infants during the first 6 months of life is sudden infant death syndrome (SIDS). In older infancy (more than 6 months old) through young adulthood, injuries are the leading cause of cardiac arrest and death. The most common causes of fatal injury in children and adolescents are motor vehicle crashes, drowning, burns and smoke inhalation, and firearms (unintentional gunshot wounds, suicide, and homicide). Children are also at risk for death or disability from poisoning and choking on toys or other objects they place in their mouth.

Although injuries are the major cause of death in children, a large variety of medical conditions also may lead to cardiac or breathing emergencies, such as asthma, diabetes, seizures, and serious infections. Children with heart conditions, respiratory (breathing) problems, or other chronic diseases may have a higher risk of cardiac arrest or serious illness requiring emergency care. If you know **when** to phone 911 (or other emergency response number) and **how** to provide rescue breathing, chest compressions, and relief of choking, your actions can be lifesaving.

The victim of an emergency, such as a child who nearly drowns, can be saved if people at the scene act quickly to create a Chain of Survival. In this chapter you will learn the critical actions that make up the 4 links in the AHA pediatric Chain of Survival. You will learn how to minimize the risk of death due to SIDS or injury, to recognize the signs of breathing emergencies (including choking or foreign-body airway obstruction), and to recognize the signs of cardiac arrest. You will learn to perform the steps of CPR and when to activate the EMS system.

The symbol of the AHA pediatric Chain of Survival **(Figure 1)** depicts the critical actions required to prevent and treat many life-threatening emergencies, including cardiac arrest and choking. The Chain of Survival provides a lifesaving progression of actions linking infants and children to the help they need. As the person responsible for the first links in the Chain of Survival, **you** link the infant or child at risk to the best chance of survival.

The first step in the Chain of Survival is to prevent the need for CPR by preventing the most common causes of injuries and cardiac arrest in infants and children. Information about *prevention* of SIDS and injuries is included in Chapter 2 of this module. Despite attempts to prevent emergencies, they still occur, and you must recognize when a serious emergency exists. When you recognize the emergency, the next 2 links — CPR and activation of the EMS system (phone 911 or other emergency response number) — are in your hands. *You* perform these actions and connect the links that increase a child's chance of survival. Skilled rescuers and emergency professionals will respond to the 911 call and provide advanced care (the fourth link in the Chain of Survival).

To save the lives of infants and children, *each set of actions or link in the Chain of Survival is essential.* If any link in the chain is weak, delayed, or missing, a child victim's chances of survival are lessened.

First Link: Prevention of Injuries and Arrest

Reducing the Risk of SIDS

SIDS is the leading cause of death in infants 1 to 6 months of age. SIDS is the sudden death of an infant, typically between the ages of 1 month and 1 year, that is not explained by the infant's medical history or other causes even when an autopsy is performed. The frequency of SIDS is much higher in infants who sleep on their stomach

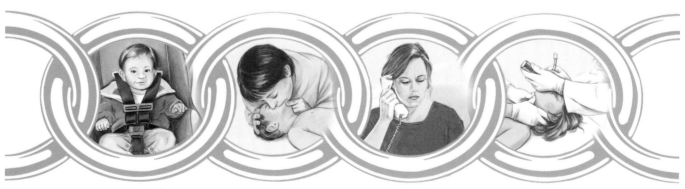

© 2000 American Heart Association

FIGURE 1.
The AHA pediatric Chain of Survival. **Link 1:** Prevention of injuries and arrest. **Link 2:** CPR. **Link 3:** Phone 911. **Link 4:** Advanced care.

than in infants who sleep on their back (supine) or side. All parents and those responsible for the care of children should be aware of the need to lay healthy infants on their back for sleeping. Chapter 2 discusses SIDS in more detail.

Preventing Injuries

Injuries are the most common cause of death in older infants, children, adolescents, young adults, and adults up to 44 years of age. One of every 3 deaths among children in the United States results from an injury. Injuries not only can cause death but also often require treatment in an Emergency Department or other medical care center. This year 1 of every 5 children will be injured seriously enough to require treatment in an Emergency Department. This means it is very likely that a child you know will be injured seriously enough this year to require emergency care. Injuries are frequently thought of as unavoidable "accidents." But at least half of fatal injuries can be prevented through simple interventions in the home, car, childcare center, school, and playground. Simple injury prevention strategies will be taught during the AHA Heartsaver CPR Course for Infant and Child.

The Safety Checklist in Chapter 2 will help you identify risks for injury at home, in the car, at childcare centers, schools, and playgrounds and will identify preventive interventions to reduce risk. It is impossible to eliminate every risk in a child's environment. For this reason young children must be closely supervised. In addition, you need to know what to do if a child in your care becomes injured or develops a breathing emergency or cardiac arrest.

Second Link: CPR

To perform CPR correctly you must first recognize the signs of an emergency. Signs of emergencies are described in more detail in Chapter 3. You must recognize the signs of serious breathing problems (including choking) and cardiac arrest. *Any infant or child* who suddenly becomes *unresponsive* should receive emergency care. An "unresponsive" infant or child has no reaction when you speak loudly and gently tap him. Cardiac arrest, choking, head injury, and poisoning can cause a victim to become unresponsive. Although many other conditions can cause a victim to be unresponsive, *all* unresponsive victims will benefit from activation of the Chain of Survival.

CPR is a set of actions that the rescuer performs in sequence to *assess and support* the airway, breathing, and circulation. CPR is performed in steps **(see Figure 2)** so that the rescuer provides only the support the victim needs. CPR may restore breathing to a child who has stopped breathing, and it will also buy time by maintaining oxygen flow to the heart and brain until more advanced care can be provided. Infants and children who suffer out-of-hospital respiratory arrest and cardiac arrest but receive immediate CPR from bystanders have a much higher rate of survival than those who do not receive this support.

FIGURE 2.
The steps of infant and child CPR. CPR includes both assessment and support steps, performed in sequence. The rescuer provides only the support that the victim needs.

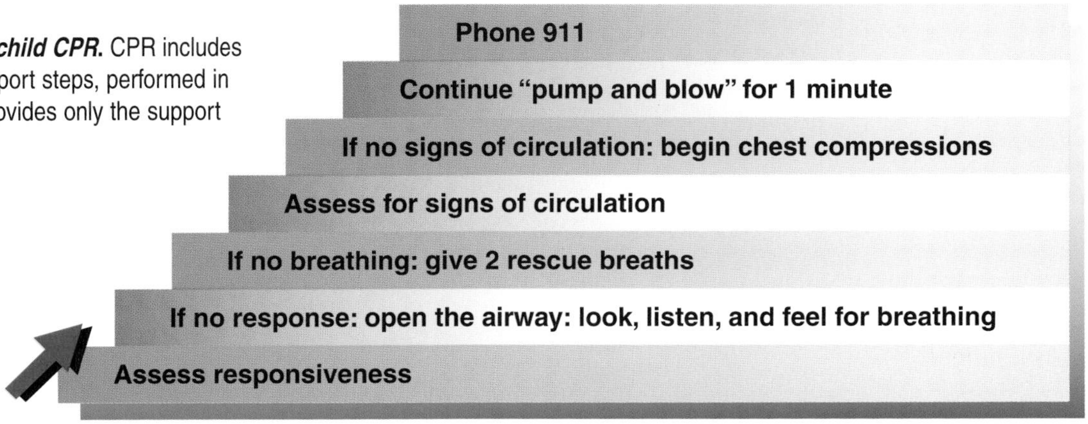

Phone 911

Continue "pump and blow" for 1 minute

If no signs of circulation: begin chest compressions

Assess for signs of circulation

If no breathing: give 2 rescue breaths

If no response: open the airway: look, listen, and feel for breathing

Assess responsiveness

"Call First" Versus "Call Fast": Heart Disease in Children, Cardiac Emergencies, and Public Access Defibrillation

Most life-threatening emergencies in infants and children are caused by breathing difficulties, and the victim will benefit from immediate CPR. For this reason the AHA recommends that if you are alone, provide approximately 1 minute of CPR *before* you leave the victim to phone 911 or other emergency response number.

Sudden cardiac arrest in infants and children may occasionally be caused by an abnormal heart rhythm (arrhythmia) that prevents the heart from beating effectively. Many serious arrhythmias must be treated by delivery of a shock to the heart. A shock that converts VF to a perfusing rhythm is called **defibrillation**. If defibrillation is needed, it must be provided within a few minutes after the onset of arrest to be effective. If a child's doctor or nurse determines that a child is at high risk for arrhythmias and cardiac arrest, the child's parents and primary caregivers (teachers, daycare providers, babysitters) should be notified. If the child is at high risk, the doctor or nurse will recommend that you phone 911 **first** and then begin CPR if the child becomes unresponsive. This will ensure that trained rescuers will arrive quickly with a defibrillator (see also Appendix C, Special Resuscitation Situations).

The AHA has developed a public health initiative to promote rapid defibrillation of *adult* victims of cardiac arrest (including children 8 years of age and older) in the out-of-hospital setting. This public health initiative is called *public access defibrillation* (PAD). In PAD programs highly accurate, computerized devices called *automated external defibrillators* (AEDs) are available for use by trained rescuers throughout the community, particularly in locations where many people gather. In an emergency, PAD program AEDs are quickly available for use by police officers, firefighters, airline personnel, security guards, and trained lay rescuers. They may be placed at worksites, public places such as sports arenas, airports, and even on airplanes. AEDs are designed for use in sudden cardiac arrest in adults. **At present AEDs should *not* be used for infants or children less than 8 years old.**

Third Link: Phone 911

An EMS system is a community-wide, coordinated means of responding to sudden illness or injury. It is a complete rescue system. An effective EMS system has many elements. You must understand how to access the system by phoning 911 or the emergency response number in your area.

After completing this course you should be able to recognize the warning signs of breathing emergencies (including choking) and cardiac arrest in infants and children. You should also be able to provide immediate emergency care to sustain life (CPR) until EMS personnel arrive.

As soon as you recognize an emergency involving an infant or child, shout for help and begin CPR *immediately*. If a second rescuer is present, send that rescuer to phone 911. If you are alone, complete your assessment, provide approximately 1 minute of CPR if needed, and then phone 911.

Lay responders often serve as part of an emergency response system in the workplace. If the emergency response system includes an emergency number other than 911, you should use that number as instructed. Operators who answer this emergency response number should determine your location and the nature of the emergency, call the local EMS service, and send other trained rescuers who are on-site to help you until EMS personnel arrive. If you are part of a workplace emergency response system, you should phone the emergency response number in your workplace whenever this manual indicates that you should phone 911.

When you telephone for help, the dispatcher will ask you questions. The information you provide to the dispatcher will be relayed to a response team. Answer in short sentences, giving only the requested information, and follow any instructions the dispatcher gives. The dispatcher will ask questions such as

- **"What is your emergency?"** You might answer, *"A child was just pulled out of the lake. He is limp and blue."*
- **"What's happening now?"** *"My friend is giving CPR."*
- **"Where is the victim located?"** *"We're at Lake Union, the north beach, near the boat dock."*
- **"What number are you calling from?"** *"555-1313."*

At this point the dispatcher may give you directions such as **"Stay on the line until I tell you to hang up. Rescuers are being sent to your location. Please send someone to meet them and direct them to the scene."** The dispatcher may also tell you how to perform CPR. You may then perform CPR with the guidance of the dispatcher or relay the dispatcher's instructions to other rescuers (see FYI... Emergency Medical Dispatch Assistance and Enhanced 911 at right).

Case Scenario Question: What information could you give to an EMS dispatcher about the child pulled from the water in the case scenario at the beginning of the chapter? What additional information should you have when you phone 911?

Fourth Link: Advanced Care

The fourth link in the Chain of Survival is early advanced care. Highly trained EMS personnel called *emergency medical technicians* (EMTs) provide CPR and defibrillation. Paramedics also provide CPR and defibrillation as well as more advanced care, such as administration of cardiac drugs and placement of breathing tubes. These advanced actions help the heart start beating effectively and preserve functioning of the vital organs. EMS personnel also rapidly and safely transport the child to a facility where ongoing care can be delivered.

FYI...

Emergency Medical Dispatch Assistance and Enhanced 911

In many areas of the United States EMDs are taught how to help callers give emergency care. The EMD can coach you through the basic steps of CPR. If you can bring the phone to the victim's side, follow the dispatcher's instructions. If other rescuers are at the scene and the EMD provides instructions, stay on the phone and do the following:

- Repeat the dispatcher's instructions loudly to the other rescuers and confirm that they are following each step.
- If the victim vomits or other complications occur, tell the dispatcher. No one is expected to perform perfectly in such a crisis.
- Be sure that rescuers follow each instruction, even if it takes extra seconds.
- Ensure the safety of the rescuer at all times.
- When EMS personnel arrive at the victim's side, the dispatcher will hang up after confirming the arrival of EMS personnel.
- You hang up last or if instructed to do so by the dispatcher.

Find out if your community has *enhanced* 911. In enhanced 911 systems a computer automatically confirms the caller's address. This allows the dispatcher to locate the caller even if the caller is unable to speak or the connection is broken. If your community does not have an enhanced 911 system, you should become a vocal advocate for such services in your community. Enhanced 911 can save precious seconds, minutes, and lives.

Case Scenario Note: Victims of submersion require immediate CPR and early advanced life support, particularly support of breathing. It is important to initiate CPR immediately after the victim is pulled from the water and notify 911 as soon as possible. If you are alone, give approximately 1 minute of CPR, then phone 911 to ensure that EMS personnel arrive quickly.

How to Recognize Life-Threatening Emergencies

- Breathing Emergencies
- Respiratory Arrest
- Cardiac Arrest
- Choking

How to Recognize Breathing Emergencies

In children breathing emergencies can lead to cardiac arrest. Breathing emergencies can be characterized by *increased* or *decreased* breathing effort. Choking, croup (a viral infection causing a hoarse cough), asthma, serious pneumonia, or submersion (near-drowning) may cause *increased* breathing effort. A child with any of these conditions is struggling to breathe and may be breathing rapidly. The rescuer will need to decide whether the child's breathing is resulting in *poor* air exchange, which requires emergency treatment, or *good* air exchange, which provides sufficient air movement and does not require emergency treatment.

Signs of *poor* air exchange include a weak cry, inability to speak or a weak voice, decreasing alertness or responsiveness, and blue or pale lips and tongue. If you observe these signs, **activate the EMS system** and make sure that the airway is open.

Children with *decreased* breathing effort breathe at a very slow rate or very shallowly. They cannot maintain enough oxygen in the blood. If this condition is not corrected, it can lead to respiratory or cardiac arrest. Head injury, drug intoxication, and a host of serious medical conditions that can affect the breathing control center of the brain can cause decreased breathing effort. Children with decreased breathing effort require rescue breathing and emergency treatment.

Critical Concepts

Signs of a Breathing Emergency With Poor Air Exchange — Signals to Phone 911 (or other emergency response number)

- Weak cry
- Inability to speak or a weak voice
- Decreasing alertness or responsiveness
- Blue or pale lips and tongue
- Very rapid breathing with evidence that the infant or child is working hard to breathe OR
- Very slow, shallow breathing (infant or child is barely breathing)

How to Recognize Respiratory Arrest

Respiratory arrest is present when the infant or child is not breathing at all or is breathing so slowly, shallowly, or irregularly that oxygenation of the blood cannot occur. The term *respiratory arrest* is used for infants and children who are not breathing effectively but who still have signs of circulation. You can determine that respiratory arrest has occurred only as you go through the steps of CPR. A child in respiratory arrest will be unresponsive. Open the airway and look, listen, and feel for breathing. You will observe no breathing or only occasional or very shallow breathing effort. Provide 2 breaths, watching the chest to see if it rises with each breath. The child in respiratory arrest will demonstrate signs of circulation (breathing, coughing, or movement in response to the rescue breaths), confirming that the child has spontaneous blood flow (circulation); this child does not have cardiac arrest. However, the child will not have normal, effective breathing (respiratory arrest is present).

How to Recognize Cardiac Arrest

In children cardiac arrest (also called "cardiopulmonary arrest") may result from a large number of conditions. Cardiac arrest means that the infant or child is unresponsive, not breathing,

Critical Concepts

Causes of Cardiac Arrest —
Differences Between Infants and Children and Adults

Infants and Children	Adults
■ Often caused by breathing emergencies	■ Usually caused by abnormal heart rhythm
■ Onset often follows illness or injury	■ Onset is often sudden
■ Primary heart rhythm problems are uncommon, especially in children less than 8 years old	■ Breathing emergencies are less common than sudden cardiac arrest

and has no signs of circulation. Cardiac arrest in infants and children is most often caused by breathing emergencies, SIDS, or injuries. Cardiac arrest may also result from an abnormal heart rhythm, particularly if the child has a heart disease.

You must remember that an unresponsive child may be in cardiac arrest. An unresponsive child is a red flag for an emergency: Act immediately!

Provide CPR for any child who is unresponsive. The earlier you provide CPR, the greater the child's chance of survival. CPR consists of 3 basic steps known as the *ABCs of CPR* because they address 3 areas: **A**irway, **B**reathing, and **C**irculation. At each step you must *assess* that component and then provide the support the victim requires. CPR keeps oxygen-containing blood flowing to the brain and heart until defibrillation, medications, insertion of a breathing tube, or other advanced care can restore normal heart action. The steps of CPR are described in more detail in Chapter 3.

The child in cardiac arrest *shows no response, has no normal breathing, and has no signs of circulation.*

1. No response: The child appears limp and does not respond to voice or touch. If the child does not respond, shout for help. If a second rescuer is available, send that person to phone 911 (or other emergency response number) to

activate the EMS system. If you are alone, perform the steps of CPR for about 1 minute and then leave the victim to phone 911. Once you determine that the child is unresponsive and shout for help, open the airway and assess breathing.

2. No normal breathing: While holding the child's airway open, *look, listen, and feel* for breathing. If the child does not breathe for several seconds, provide 2 rescue breaths. Each breath must make the chest rise.

3. No signs of circulation: Signs of circulation include normal breathing, coughing, or movement in response to the 2 rescue breaths. If no signs of circulation are present, the child will not breathe, cough, or move after you provide the 2 rescue breaths. Signs of circulation are present if there is adequate oxygenation and cardiac function to deliver blood to the brain and body. If no signs of circulation are present, the child is probably in cardiac arrest and requires rapid intervention to restore circulation and breathing.

You can confirm that the infant or child is in cardiac arrest only *after* you have delivered 2 breaths. If the child has no signs of circulation (breathing, coughing, or movement) after delivery of the 2 rescue breaths, begin chest compressions. Provide chest compressions and rescue breaths (ventilations) at a ratio of 5 to 1 (5 compressions for every rescue breath).

A child who does respond to the 2 rescue breaths may be in respiratory arrest but is not in cardiac arrest. A child in *respiratory arrest* is not breathing effectively but is responsive to the rescue breaths you provide (signs of circulation are present).

Case Scenario Question: Could the child in the case scenario at the beginning of this chapter be in cardiac arrest? The child was pulled from the water, and he is limp and has blue lips. How would you assess the child to determine whether cardiac arrest has occurred?

How to Recognize Severe or Complete Foreign-Body Airway Obstruction (Choking)

Choking is a common cause of preventable death in children. Infants and children can choke on pieces of food, toys, or any other item small enough to fit in their mouth. You can prevent choking in the following ways:

- Do not allow children to play, walk, cry, or run with anything in their mouth.
- Serve infants and children food that is appropriate for their age and size. Keep seeds, nuts, popcorn, and small hard candies away from children less than 4 years old.
- Keep foreign objects such as marbles, beads, and thumbtacks away from infants and small children. A useful rule of thumb is to prevent young children from playing with toys or other items that are small enough to fit through the tube of a roll of toilet paper.

To treat a victim of choking, **you must recognize the signs of severe or complete foreign-body airway obstruction and act quickly to remove the obstruction.** If *severe or complete* obstruction of the airway has occurred, no air can pass the obstruction, so the child will be *unable to make sounds, cough forcefully, speak,*

Critical Concepts

Signs of Severe or Complete Airway Obstruction in Infants and Children

- Universal sign of choking (clutches neck)
- Child unable to speak or makes only faint sounds
- Weak, ineffective coughs
- High-pitched sounds or no sounds while inhaling
- Increased difficulty breathing
- Blue lips or skin (cyanosis)
- If the obstruction is not relieved, the child becomes unresponsive

or cry out loud. An older child may use the "universal sign of choking" (clutching the neck). The child may nod if you ask if he is choking and may shake his head if you ask if he can speak.

If a foreign object causes *severe or complete* airway obstruction, you must remove the object immediately. Otherwise the child may become unresponsive, and cardiac arrest may develop.

*If a child is coughing vigorously and producing a loud sound, the airway is only partially obstructed. In such a case do **not** attempt to relieve the obstruction.* As long as the child is able to speak or cough loudly and remains responsive, do not interfere but take the child to a physician or medical center. Phone 911 if the child is in distress.

If you are not sure whether the child has severe or complete airway obstruction but the child's cough seems weak, the child is very agitated, or you have another concern about the child's ability to breathe, phone 911 and try to keep the child calm until EMS personnel arrive. *Do not drive a child with these clinical signs to the hospital because you will be unable to provide care while driving.*

Summary

The goal of this course is to provide you with the knowledge and skills to prevent cardiac arrest by preventing SIDS and common injuries, to recognize cardiac and breathing emergencies, and to begin CPR. You will also learn when and how to activate the EMS system.

Prevention of common causes of cardiac arrest, particularly SIDS and injury, is the first link in the AHA pediatric Chain of Survival. The second link in the chain is provision of CPR. If a second rescuer is present, that rescuer can complete the third link in the chain, phone 911 while you perform CPR. If you are alone during an emergency, phone 911 after providing approximately 1 minute of CPR. These are important steps that you will practice many times during this course. The fourth link in the Chain of Survival, advanced care, is provided by EMS and hospital personnel.

The knowledge and skills you learn in this course will make you a vital part of your community's Chain of Survival for infants and children, and we encourage you to put what you learn to good use. Following are a few things you can do:

- Prevent cardiac arrest by reducing the risk of SIDS in infants and injury in infants and children.
- Share this information with your family, friends, and coworkers.
- Know the signs of breathing emergencies (including severe or complete choking) and cardiac arrest and respond as soon as you recognize them.
- Know the steps of CPR and do not hesitate to use them in an emergency.
- Know when to phone 911, answer the dispatcher's questions to the best of your ability, and follow the dispatcher's instructions.

Learning Checklist

Take a moment to review the key information you learned in this chapter:

✔ The 4 links in the AHA pediatric Chain of Survival are

- Prevent injuries and arrest
- CPR
- Phone 911 (or other emergency response number)
- Advanced care

✔ Signs of a breathing emergency with poor air exchange are

- Weak cry
- Inability to speak or a weak voice
- Decreasing responsiveness
- Blue or pale lips and tongue
- Very rapid breathing with evidence that the child is working hard to breathe **or** very slow, shallow breathing (child is barely breathing)

✔ A child with severe or complete foreign-body airway obstruction will often demonstrate the following:

- Universal sign of choking (clutching the neck)
- Inability to make a sound (the child cannot speak, cough forcefully, or cry) or will be able to make only very weak sounds
- Weak, ineffective coughs
- High-pitched sounds or no sounds while inhaling
- Increased difficulty breathing
- May become blue if the obstruction is not relieved
- May become unresponsive if the obstruction is not relieved

✔ The 3 signs of cardiac arrest in an infant or child are

- No response to voice or touch
- No normal breathing
- No signs of circulation

Review Questions

1. **A 6-year-old boy collapses in your presence while you are caring for him. After prevention, what is the next link in the Chain of Survival for unresponsive infants and children?**

   a. phone 911 or other emergency response number

   b. begin CPR

   c. perform rescue breathing

   d. transfer to advanced care

2. **During a visit to the school cafeteria you observe a 4-year-old girl in distress, which you suspect may be related to choking. Which of the following signs indicate severe or complete foreign-body airway obstruction in a child?**

   a. the child can cough loudly and speak

   b. the child is breathing quietly and the lips are pink

   c. the child cannot speak, cry, or cough

   d. the child wheezes when breathing in but can speak and cough

3. **You are asked to give a lecture on emergency cardiovascular care to your local Girl Scout troop. You decide to use the Chain of Survival to illustrate the importance of preparation. What is the correct order of the links in the Chain of Survival for infants and children?**

   a. phone 911, provide CPR, provide advanced care, prevent injuries and arrest

   b. prevent infection, phone 911, provide CPR, provide advanced care

   c. provide CPR, phone 911, prevent injuries and arrest, provide advanced care

   d. prevent injuries and arrest, provide CPR, phone 911, provide advanced care

4. **While working out at your local gym, you see a 2-year-old-boy collapse. The child is unresponsive. As you perform the assessment and support steps of CPR, which of the following are the *red flags* of cardiac arrest?**

   a. the child suddenly becomes unresponsive and the lips are blue

   b. the child stiffens and then has a seizure

   c. the child has no response, no normal breathing, and no signs of circulation

   d. the child has severe difficulty breathing and is unable to cry or speak

5. **You are a daycare worker who must decide when and when not to call 911. Which of the following signs would most likely be caused by a breathing emergency and would require you to phone 911?**

   a. weak voice and cough in a child who is responsive but very sleepy and who is breathing rapidly and shallowly with blue skin or lips

   b. a loud hoarse cough in an infant who is alert and smiling

   c. rapid breathing in a child who has a fever and is speaking normally

   d. deep, regular breaths in a child who is sound asleep

6. **You are asked to phone 911 for an infant who has stopped breathing. Another rescuer is performing CPR. Which of the following most accurately summarizes the interaction you should have with the dispatcher?**

   a. tell the dispatcher to send someone as soon as possible and then hang up and go back to help the infant

   b. tell the dispatcher what happened and where you are located and then leave the phone off the hook so the call can be traced and the address can be confirmed

   c. tell the dispatcher what happened and then answer the dispatcher's questions and stay on the phone until the dispatcher tells you to hang up

   d. tell the dispatcher that you don't have time to answer all of her questions and that she should just send someone right away

How did you do?

1, b; **2,** c; **3,** d; **4,** c; **5,** a; **6,** c.

Module 2

Chapter **2**

Prevention of Injuries and Arrest
Infant and Child Safety

Case Scenario 1

You are responding to a call for help on the beach. A child has just been pulled from the water and appears limp.

What is the cause of this emergency? Could it have been prevented? How?

Case Scenario 2

You are working in a shopping mall. You hear a mother shout for help because her 3-year-old child fell down a tall flight of concrete stairs. The child is lying on the ground at the bottom of the stairs and is not moving. The child is limp and does not respond to your touch or voice. The mother is crying and asking for your help because she doesn't know what to do.

What should you do first? What should you tell the mother to do? Is this a common cause of a life-threatening breathing emergency in children? How could this emergency have been prevented? How should you assess and support this child?

Learning Objectives

After reading this chapter you should be able to

1. Name the most common cause of death in infants from birth to 6 months of age.
2. Describe the sleeping positions that will reduce the infant's risk of SIDS.
3. List the 5 most common causes of fatal injury in infants and children.
4. Describe how to safely secure an infant and a child up to 12 years of age in a car.
5. Describe ways to prevent injuries indoors.
6. Describe ways to prevent injuries outdoors.

Reducing the Risk of SIDS

SIDS (sudden infant death syndrome) is the sudden death of an infant, typically between the ages of 1 month and 1 year, that is not explained by the infant's medical history or other causes even when an autopsy (postmortem examination) is performed. SIDS probably includes a variety of conditions that all result in death during sleep. It is probably caused by several mechanisms, including a form of suffocation when the infant rebreathes air while laying face down or on a fluffy comforter or blanket made of lamb's wool. Most SIDS deaths occur in the first 6 months of life, with the highest frequency occurring in infants between the ages of 2 and 4 months. Many factors are associated with an increased risk of SIDS: a prone sleeping position (on the stomach), the winter months, low family income, male gender, being a sibling of a SIDS victim, a mother who smokes or is addicted to drugs, a history of severe life-threatening events, and low birthweight.

Several years ago researchers discovered that SIDS occurred much more frequently among infants who sleep on their stomach than among infants who sleep on their back or side. Australia, New Zealand, and several European countries documented a significant reduction in the incidence of SIDS when parents and childcare providers were taught to place healthy infants on their back or side to sleep. A "Back to Sleep" public education campaign was introduced in the United States in 1992. That year approximately 7000 infants in the United States died of SIDS. In 1997, 5 years after the start of the campaign, 2991 infants died of SIDS.

All parents and anyone responsible for the care of infants should be aware of the need to lay healthy infants on their back (supine position) for sleeping. The supine sleeping position has not been associated with an increase in any significant problems, such as vomiting or aspiration. Infants may also be laid on their side, but they should be propped and positioned so they cannot roll onto their stomach. In addition, infants should not sleep on or be wrapped in soft materials such as lamb's wool or a fluffy comforter and should not sleep with objects such as stuffed animals that might trap exhaled air near the face.

Prevention of Injuries in Infants, Children, and Adolescents

The most common causes of fatal injuries in infants, children, and adolescents are motor vehicle crashes (including occupant injuries, pedestrian injuries, and bicycle-related head injuries), submersion (drowning), choking, burns or smoke inhalation, and firearms (including unintentional shootings, homicides, and suicides). Many of these injuries can be prevented if you take steps to reduce the risk of their occurring. We must all look for ways to reduce the risk of childhood injuries in homes, automobiles, schools, childcare centers, and wherever children spend time.

One of the most important elements in any child-safety program is a watchful and attentive adult. Young children require supervision; if left alone, they may get hurt. No environment is totally safe.

Motor Vehicle and Traffic Safety

Injuries sustained while riding in a car are the No. 1 preventable cause of death in young children.

A young child is very "top heavy," and the hips of a young child are difficult to anchor with a lap belt. For these reasons young children must be restrained in safety seats that secure the torso

and the hips. When children are not restrained they tend to fly headfirst through or out of the car when a collision occurs. Even in a low-speed crash an infant or small child can smash into the windshield, dashboard, or air bag with a force comparable to that of falling from a third-story window. It is *not* safe to hold a child on your lap in a car. If a crash occurs, the child will be thrown into the body of the car or crushed by your weight.

The BACK seat is the BEST seat for children *through 12 years of age.* In this location a properly restrained child is least likely to sustain injuries in a crash because the child is away from the dashboard, windshield, and front-seat air bags.

You have probably heard about injuries resulting from air bags. Air bags save lives when used "with seat belts, and they can protect drivers and passengers who are correctly "buckled up." An air bag inflates quickly and forcefully to cushion a victim during a crash. During inflation an air bag can strike anything or anyone, including children who are near the dashboard, and the impact of the air bag can cause serious head and neck injuries and even death. Air bags have saved more than 3000 lives nationwide since they were introduced, but inflation of air bags has been associated with the deaths of several children and even small adults. Most of those injured by air bags were *not* properly restrained.

To prevent injuries due to air bags, everyone riding in a car must be properly restrained, and young children (12 years old and younger) should *not* ride in the front seat if the car has a passenger-side air bag. Do not place *any* car seat in the front seat of a car with a passenger-side air bag because these seats position the child too close to the air bags. Never place rear-facing infant safety seats in the front seat of a car with a passenger-side air bag because the infant's head will be positioned very near the dashboard. If the air bag inflates, it can drive the infant seat into the automobile seat, injuring the infant's head and neck. Until "smart" passenger-side air bags are widely available, take the following precautions to reduce the risk of injury due to air bags:

- Use child-restraint devices and lap and shoulder belts appropriate for your child's age.
- For infants weighing less than 20 pounds (less than 9 kg) and less than 1 year old:
  — Use a rear-facing car seat secured in the BACK seat of the car.
  — *Never* place an infant in the front seat of a car with a passenger-side air bag.
- For children weighing more than 20 pounds (more than 9 kg) and more than 1 year old up to 4 years old:
  — Use child-restraint seats secured in the BACK seat of the car.
- For children 4 through 12 years of age:
  — For children less than 4 feet, 9 inches (less than 58 inches or 148 cm) tall and weighing less than 80 pounds (less than 36 kg), use a belt-positioning booster seat secured in the back seat.
  — Children at least 4 feet, 9 inches (at least 58 inches or 148 cm) tall and weighing at least 80 pounds (at least 36 kg) can usually be properly restrained with both a lap and shoulder belt in the BACK seat of the car. The shoulder belt should cross the shoulder down to the hip and should *not* cross the face and neck. The lap belt should fit snugly across the hips.
- For children more than 12 years old:
  — Use lap and shoulder belts (make sure the shoulder belt fits from the shoulder down to the hip and does not cross the face).
  — When children (or small adults) are seated in the front seat, move the front seat as far away from the dashboard as possible.

Critical Concepts

Automobile Passenger Safety

- EVERYONE in the car must "buckle up" with age-appropriate restraint devices.
- The BEST seat is the BACK seat for children 12 years old and younger.
  — **Never** place an infant in the front seat of a car with a passenger-side air bag.
  — **Never place** children in child-safety seats in the front seat.
  — **Use proper child-restraint devices (including belt-positioning booster seats) for children less than 4 feet 9 inches (less than 58 inches or less than 148 cm) tall and weighing less than 80 pounds (less than 36 kg).**
  — Use lap and shoulder belts for children at least 4 feet 9 inches (at least 58 inches or 148 cm) tall and at least 80 pounds or more (at least 36 kg).
  — Only adults and children older than 12 years of age should sit in the front passenger seat if the car has a passenger-side air bag.
- Never allow a child to ride in a vehicle with someone whose ability to drive may be compromised by fatigue, medications, alcohol, or drugs. If you have any doubt about the driver's safety, make other arrangements for your child's transportation.

When you secure a safety seat in an automobile, test it for tightness by pushing the seat forward, backward, and side to side. Tighten the belt to ensure that the seat does not move more than ½ inch (1 cm).

For information about children and air bags, call the National Highway Traffic Safety Administration Auto Safety Hotline toll free at 1-800-424-9393 or 1-888-327-4236. Extensive information may also be found at their website: www.nhtsa.dot.gov.

Children learn by example. Be sure that you and every person who rides with you buckles up for *every ride*. Follow the watchwords of the American Academy of Pediatrics and "Make every ride a safe ride."

Not all children who die of traffic-related injuries are passengers in cars. Some are injured or killed while walking or playing near streets or while riding a bicycle.

- Infant and toddler pedestrians are most commonly killed by cars backing out of driveways or parking lots.
- Children between the ages of 5 and 9 years risk injury or death by darting out in front of traffic while playing or crossing the street in the middle of the block. Children must be taught early in life to cross streets at inter-sections, to always stop at curbs, and to *stop, look* both ways, and *listen* for cars before crossing any street.
- Children riding bicycles can be injured when they collide with cars or fixed objects or when they are thrown from the bicycle. *The most serious bicycle-related injuries are head injuries, which can cause death or permanent brain damage. The severity of these head injuries can be reduced by about 85% if children wear bicycle helmets* approved by the Snell Memorial Foundation or the American National Standards Institute (ANSI) *every time* they ride a bicycle. The helmet must fit snugly to protect the child properly. For more information on selecting and using helmets, visit the American Academy of Pediatrics website at www.aap.org/family/thelmabt.htm.

Indoor Safety

One of the most important safety items in any area where children spend time is an emergency sticker on the telephone. This sticker should contain the telephone numbers of the police, fire department, ambulance, local hospital, physician, and poison control center in your area and your home address and telephone number. It is also worthwhile to teach young children to dial the emergency response number and to state their first and last names and address.

Choking, Strangulation, and Suffocation

Choking and suffocation are among the most common causes of preventable death in children less than 1 year old. They cause many deaths in children less than 14 years old every year. Choking occurs when food, toys, or other objects block the windpipe (trachea). Strangulation is caused by constriction about the neck. Suffocation occurs when there is blockage of the nose, mouth, or windpipe.

The most common objects that cause choking in infants and children are

- Foods such as hot dogs, grapes, nuts, popcorn, and hard candy.
- Toys or parts of toys that are small enough to place in the mouth; *infants and children should not be allowed to play with a toy that can fit through the tube in the center of a roll of toilet paper.*
- Uninflated balloons or pieces of a burst balloon (these can be particularly hard to remove).
- Other small items such as coins, marbles, buttons, beads, watch or camera batteries, and safety pins.

Strangulation of infants and children in the home is most commonly linked to

- Drapery and extension cords (tie these cords well above the floor to keep them out of the reach of small children; eliminate loops of cord within a child's reach).
- Cords from which toys and objects such as rattles, pacifiers, and jewelry are hung around the child's neck.

Suffocation in the home is linked to

- Plastic bags (carefully dispose of plastic bags such as those from the grocery store or dry cleaner so that children cannot find them and play with them).
- Laying infants on their stomach to sleep (SIDS is less likely to occur if infants are laid on their back; also do not lay infants on soft materials such as lamb's wool or a fluffy comforter and do not allow them to sleep with stuffed animals).

Burns and Smoke Inhalation

Burns and smoke inhalation are frequent causes of injury and death in children, particularly in young children. Most fire-related deaths and serious injuries are caused by smoke inhalation. *These deaths can be prevented by installing and maintaining smoke detectors on each level of your home or childcare center.* Most smoke detectors require batteries. Develop a schedule to change the batteries of the smoke detector at least twice every year (for example, change them every fall and spring when you change the time on your clocks). Every home with young children should have smoke detectors.

It is also important to keep matches away from children and to avoid smoking in bed. Electrical short circuits also may cause house fires and deaths; do not use appliances with frayed cords or damaged plugs.

Most scalds are caused by a hot liquid that spills on the child. This burn injury is usually not fatal, but it can cause long-term disability. Scalds usually occur in the

- **Kitchen:** Toddlers often grab pot handles that extend over the edge of the stove, spilling the boiling contents on themselves. Prevent these injuries by turning pot handles toward the center and back of the stove.

- **Bath:** Young children may turn on the hot water and be scalded. Water at a temperature of 140°F (60°C) causes a scald in 6 seconds; at 120°F (48.9°C) the water would probably require 5 minutes to cause a scald. To prevent scald injuries in the bathtub, check the temperature of your water heater to make sure it is set between 120°F and 130°F (48.9°C to 54.4°C). Some water heaters are preset at 150°F.

Burns also can occur when a child comes into contact with a hot iron, a curling iron, or a heat source such as a wood stove or wall heater. These burns can be prevented. Keep irons out of your child's reach and place a barrier around wood stoves, radiators, and other heat sources. Curtains, linens, and furniture should be moved well away from heaters.

Provide ventilation for kerosene and gasoline-powered heaters. They cannot be used in a closed space or closed room (carbon monoxide poisoning can develop).

Firearm Injuries

Injuries caused by firearms are a leading cause of death and disability in children, adolescents, and young adults. These injuries may be unintentional or intentional (suicide or homicide). Most firearm injuries result from handguns, and most child-related shootings involve guns obtained in the home of the child victim or a friend. Guns in the home are often loaded and readily accessible to children (for example, under a pillow or in a drawer).

If you keep a gun in your home, ensure that the gun *cannot* be operated by unsupervised children. Store the gun unloaded in a locked cabinet or drawer, and store the ammunition in a separate location. Trigger locks or lockboxes should be used to secure every firearm in homes where children visit or live. Check the guns daily to ensure that children have not touched them, played with them, or taken them to school.

Poisoning

Poisoning is common in children. More than 250,000 household products are available today, and many contain harmful chemicals. Many adults have miniature drugstores at home, even in desk drawers and nightstands. It is not surprising that children, who are curious about everything, are often victims of poisoning.

Some common poisons found in the home are

- Prescription and nonprescription medications, particularly iron pills, vitamins containing iron, acetaminophen (such as Tylenol), and aspirin
- Plants
- Cleansers, polishing agents, ammonia, and detergents
- Cosmetics and hair care products (for example, hair-coloring agents)
- Alcohol and liquor
- Insect and rodent poisons and moth balls
- Gasoline, kerosene, and other petroleum products
- Pesticides, weed killers, and fertilizers
- Lye and acids
- Paint and paint thinners

The best place to obtain information about poisons is your regional poison control center. The staff can quickly provide accurate and up-to-date information about almost any poisonous or potentially poisonous product. They will also provide immediate first aid instructions and recommendations for treatment. This service is available 24 hours a day. Write the telephone number of the nearest poison control center on the sticker that you post near your telephone. In an emergency, however, you should phone 911.

Syrup of ipecac (a substance that causes vomiting) was previously recommended to reduce drug absorption after ingestion of a poison. Treatment with syrup of ipecac is often *not* helpful, particularly if the child is within 15 minutes of medical care. It may even be harmful to induce vomiting after ingestion of some toxic substances. **Always** check with the poison control center or your physician before giving syrup of ipecac.

To prevent poisoning, store medicines, vitamins, and household cleaning products in areas inaccessible to small children. Never store poisons in empty food or drink containers (eg, *do not* store kerosene in soda bottles). Poisons should be stored in specially designed and labeled containers in high places out of a child's sight and reach. A high, locked cabinet is the best place to store poisons. Remember that resourceful children can stack objects and climb to reach toxic items stored on high shelves.

Check prescription and over-the-counter medications at least annually, and destroy all medications that are past their expiration date by flushing them down the toilet. Do not throw expired or unneeded medications in the garbage; young children may find them.

Falls

Falls are commonplace and often minor, but they are the most frequent cause of injury in children less than 6 years old. About 200 children die as a result of falls each year. Infants and children may be injured by

- Falls out of sinks or bathtubs or off countertops or changing tables.
- Climbing out of a crib.
- Falls down stairs. Twenty percent of all falls occur on stairs. Keep stairways as safe as possible by providing adequate lighting, removing toys, tacking down loose carpet, and using appropriate gate enclosures.

Avoid the accordion-type gates with wide gaps at the top. Instead use a safety gate that is permanently mounted or firmly attached to the wall with double closures that cannot be operated by children.

- Falls associated with infant walkers, especially near stairs or ramps.
- Falls from upper-floor windows. Open windows only from the top or 4 to 5 inches from the bottom and secure them at the proper height with a burglar lock (available at hardware stores). Place gates over the lower portion of windows in high-rise buildings.
- Falls from trees or play equipment.

Drowning Indoors

Drowning is a major cause of death and disability in children, and it occurs indoors as well as outdoors. The household bath is the most common site for drowning in infants up to 1 year of age; young children can drown in only a few inches of water. Always closely supervise infants, toddlers, and preschoolers in the bath or near any container of water, including buckets and toilets. Keep toilet lids closed, and do not allow infants or toddlers to play near industrial-size buckets (5 gallons or larger) containing liquids. Because young children have large, heavy heads, if they lean over and fall into a bucket or any large liquid container, their legs may be too light and their arms too weak to lift their heads out of the water.

Outdoor Safety

When children play outdoors they will be active. You can prevent injuries by following some simple safety guidelines.

Most important, children should play away from streets. This eliminates the temptation to follow a ball or other toy into the street. Toddlers playing outside should always be supervised, and young children playing near animals must always be with an adult.

Drowning Outdoors

Drowning in backyard swimming pools is a leading cause of death and permanent brain damage in children, particularly among children 1 to 4 years of age. The natural curiosity of toddlers, their inability to appreciate the danger and depth of water, and the attraction of water play can be a dangerous combination. The young child is capable of getting into a swimming pool alone but may be incapable of getting out. **No child is "drownproof,"** and the ability to swim does *not* prevent drowning.

Do not allow children to have unsupervised access to swimming pools. All pools, hot tubs, and spas should be completely surrounded by a nonclimbable fence at least 5 feet high with a self-closing, self-latching gate. Do *not* consider the house to be part of the fence because toddlers may leave the house and go to the pool area. Pool covers and alarms may give a false sense of security because they will not prevent drowning. Contrary to popular belief, the drowning child often sinks quietly without screaming for help or thrashing, so the child may never activate a pool alarm.

Children should **always** be supervised when they play in or around water, and all toys should be removed from the pool area at the end of every supervised swim period so that children are not lured back into the water. Parents and older children who live in a home with a swimming pool should learn CPR.

Children should wear life vests when they play on docks or at beaches or rivers. Children swimming in moving water should wear approved flotation devices. *Do not allow any child to swim alone.*

Death due to drowning in natural waters is *most frequent in adolescent boys.* It is difficult to closely observe these children, but you can still help prevent drowning by understanding why adolescents are at risk. Adolescents are risk-takers, and they are susceptible to peer pressure. These factors may cause adolescents to try to swim farther than they are capable of swimming or to swim in dangerous waters.

Playground Injuries

Children are frequently injured at the playground. Although playground injuries are not often fatal, they are common and can require medical care or hospitalization. The number and severity of these injuries can be reduced if we ensure that all playground equipment is safe. Attachments, cables, and seats of swings should be inspected regularly, particularly at the beginning and middle of every summer, and kept in good condition. Playgrounds should be built on several (4 to 6) inches of an energy-absorbing surface, such as sand, wood chips, or rubber padding. Concrete and grass do not provide adequate cushioning for children when they fall.

Safety Checklist

The checklist at the end of this chapter was developed to help you make a child's daily environment as safe as possible. It is based on the most up-to-date information on injuries and is designed to guide you through an inspection of your home, childcare center, school, babysitter's home, or wherever children spend time. Take it with you on your inspection tour, and note areas that need correction. You may be surprised to detect several potential dangers that you can remedy. You can help prevent injury and death in the children around you by following the recommendations of your course instructor and those in the checklist.

Summary

One important goal of the Heartsaver CPR Course for children and infants is to teach you a number of simple interventions that reduce the risk of arrest and serious injury in children.

Foundation Facts

Safety Supplies for Areas Where Children Live and Play

- Emergency telephone numbers posted by the phone for quick reference in case of an emergency
- A smoke detector with a working battery, mounted on the ceiling outside rooms where children play and sleep
- Trigger locks or lockboxes for firearms
- Plastic plug covers for electric outlets to protect children from electric shock
- Plastic outlet covers to use when an electrical cord is plugged into the outlet
- Cabinet latches and locks to keep children away from dangerous items such as medicines, cleaning products, and knives
- A hot water gauge (such as a meat or candy thermometer) for measuring the temperature of tap water to prevent scalding
- An out-of-reach hook-and-eye latch to prevent children from entering the basement or garage, where dangerous products are often stored

These safety devices will help reduce injuries and give you the satisfaction of knowing that you have taken steps to improve the safety of your child's environment.

Place healthy infants to sleep on their back or propped on their side to reduce the risk of SIDS. Do not lay the infant prone or on fluffy comforters or lamb's wool blankets.

Properly secure children in car seats that are correctly positioned and secured in the back seat of the car. Ensure that your children wear bicycle helmets, and teach them how to cross the street safely. To reduce injuries inside your home, childcare center, and other locations frequented by children, keep small objects out of a child's reach and do not let a child eat and run at the same time. Also, ensure that smoke detectors are working, take simple safety precautions in the kitchen, adjust the temperature of the water heater to 120° to 130°F (48.9° to 54.4°C), and watch infants and young children while they bathe. Store all poisons and firearms in a locked location away from children.

Outdoor safety requires knowledge of the risks of drowning of both small children and adolescents. Check your local playground to ensure that it is safe. Finally, use the Safety Checklist to help you remember what to look for and how to prevent injury.

Learning Checklist

Take a moment to review the key information you have learned in this chapter before evaluating your knowledge.

✔ Injury due to motor vehicle accidents is the leading cause of death in infants and children.

- All passengers should wear age-appropriate restraint devices.
- Proper restraint of children in the car is the most important preventive intervention.
- The BACK seat is the BEST seat for children 12 years old or younger.
- Never place an infant (rear-facing) car seat in the front seat of a car with a passenger-side air bag.
- Properly secure car seats following the manufacturer's installation instructions.

✔ **Fatal bicycle injuries most often result from head injury.**

- Collisions with motor vehicles and falls from bicycles cause serious injuries.
- Bicycle helmets will prevent most bicycle-related head injuries.

✔ **Drowning is the second most common cause of injury-related death in children 1 to 4 years of age.** Drowning occurs not only in pools and open bodies of water but also in bathtubs and buckets. Always watch toddlers in the bath, and be sure to empty buckets of water.

- Drowning is most common in 2 age groups: toddlers (1 to 4 years) and adolescent boys.
- Pool covers and alarms are not foolproof. Pools should be surrounded by a fence on all sides, and gates should be self-closing and self-latching.
- Adolescents have a higher risk of drowning because they like to take risks, they do not like to use safety equipment, and they will sometimes use alcohol or drugs while swimming or boating.

✔ Keep small objects away from children to reduce the risk of choking. Do not allow children to play and eat at the same time. Do not allow young children to play with toys that are small enough to fit through the tube of a roll of toilet paper.

✔ Prevent burns and smoke inhalation by taking these simple precautions:

- Check smoke detectors monthly and replace batteries twice a year.
- Keep pots and other hot items out of the reach of toddlers.
- Set the temperature of your water heater at 120°F to 130°F (48.9°C to 54.4°C).
- Check electrical cords for fraying, and cover all plugs and receptacles.

✔ Store firearms locked and unloaded and out of the reach of children.

✔ Keep medicines and household toxins out of the reach of children, inside cabinets secured with childproof latches.

Review Questions

1. **You are driving your 9-month-old niece to the store. Where should you place the car seat of an infant (up to 1 year old) in an automobile?**

   a. secure the car seat next to you while driving

   b. place the car seat in the rear center seat facing backward

   c. place the car seat facing forward when the infant is more than 6 months old and can sit unsupported

   d. secure the car seat using only the lap belt

2. **What is the correct method of securing an infant car seat in the car?**

   a. secure the car seat loosely so that the seat moves freely within the lap and shoulder belt

   b. keep the front seat close to the dashboard to prevent too much movement in a crash

   c. secure the car seat in the back seat so that it does not move

   d. secure the car seat using only the lap belt

3. **You are trying to childproof your home. Which of the following statements is true about choking and strangling?**

   a. choking and strangling do not cause death in children

   b. choking and strangling can be prevented by not allowing children to play with toys or objects that will fit through the center of a roll of toilet paper

   c. choking and strangling occur only in the home

   d. choking and strangling occur only during infancy and childhood

4. **You are babysitting 2 young children at the local pool. Effective prevention of drowning includes**

   a. always watching children in or around water

   b. using water wings while swimming

   c. keeping life preservers in a locker on the boat

   d. letting a 5-year-old watch an infant in the bathtub

5. **You have purchased a bicycle for your young son. The most effective device to reduce bicycle-related injuries is**

   a. a safety helmet

   b. bike reflectors

   c. training wheels

   d. wrist and knee pads

6. **To make your home safe in the event of an emergency, you should include all the following information on a sticker placed on or beside your phone except**

   a. telephone numbers for the EMS system, police, and fire department

   b. telephone numbers for the local hospital and poison control center

   c. social security number for each of your children

   d. your home telephone number

How did you do?

1, b; **2,** c; **3,** b; **4,** a; **5,** a; **6,** c.

Safety Checklist

This Safety Checklist was designed to help you make your home or work environment as safe as possible for infants and children. It can be used to inspect your home, the childcare center where your children stay after school, or any other place where children spend time. Take time to go around your house and see just how safe your home is for a child and learn how you can make it safer.

If you already follow the suggested safety precaution, check the box in the first column. If you need to purchase a certain item to make your home safer, the box on the far right will be shaded, indicating the need to purchase a "Safety Item." Check the shaded box when you have purchased the appropriate safety items.

	I follow this safety precaution (✔ = yes)	Purchase of safety item is required for all shaded boxes (✔ = item purchased)
Car Safety		
1. Ensure that every person in the car "buckles up" correctly.		
2. Have children less than 12 years old ride in the BACK seat with appropriate child restraints or lap-shoulder restraints.		
3. Use a rear-facing infant safety seat until infants weigh at least 20 lb and are 1 year old. ■ Secure all car seats in the BACK seat of the car. ■ Secure the seat following the manufacturer's instructions. ■ Test for tightness by pushing the seat forward, backward, and side to side. Tighten the belt to ensure that the seat does not move more than ½ inch (1 cm). ■ For proper adjustment, the seat belt buckle and latch plate (if needed) must be located well below the frame or toward the center of the seat.		☐ **Safety item — infant safety seat**
4. Wait until a child weighs 20 lb (9 kg) and is at least 1 year old and can sit with good head control before using a convertible seat or toddler seat in the forward-facing position. Place these seats in the BACK seat of the car.		☐ **Safety item — child safety seat**
5. Use a belt-positioning booster seat for children weighing 40 to 80 lb (18 to 36 kg). Secure the seat with a 3-point seat belt (lap and shoulder belt) in the BACK seat of the car. ■ If a shield is provided, fasten it close to the child's body. ■ Properly install the tether harness if required.		☐ **Safety item — belt-positioning booster seat**

	I follow this safety precaution (✓ = yes)	Purchase of safety item is required for all shaded boxes (✓ = item purchased)
Car Safety (continued)		
6. Children cannot be properly restrained with a lap-shoulder belt until they are at least 4 feet 9 inches (58 inches or 148 cm) tall, weigh 80 lb (36 kg), and can sit in the automobile seat with their knees bent over the edge. Always use a combination lap-shoulder belt to restrain children sitting in an automobile seat. ■ The shoulder belt should fit across the shoulder and breastbone. If it crosses the face and neck, use a belt-positioning booster seat to ensure that the belt is properly placed. Do not hook the shoulder belt under the child's arm. ■ All children 12 years old or younger should ride in the BACK seat.		
General Indoor Safety		
7. Place a sticker with emergency telephone numbers near or on the telephone. Include numbers for the EMS system, police, fire department, local hospital or physician, the poison control center in your area, and your telephone number.		☐ **Safety item — phone sticker with emergency response numbers**
8. Install smoke detectors on the ceiling in the hallway outside sleeping or napping areas and on each floor at the head of stairs. Test the alarm monthly and replace batteries twice a year (for example, in the fall and spring when the time changes to and from daylight saving time).		☐ **Safety item — smoke detector**
9. Ensure that there are 2 unobstructed emergency exits from the home, childcare center, classroom, or other facility where children are likely to be present.		
10. Develop and practice a fire escape plan.		
11. Ensure that a working fire extinguisher is on the premises.		☐ **Safety item — fire extinguisher**
12. All space heaters are approved; in safe condition; out of a child's reach; placed at least 3 feet from curtains, papers, and furniture; and have protective covers.		
13. All wood-burning stoves are inspected yearly and vented properly. Place stoves out of a child's reach.		

	I follow this safety precaution (✔ = yes)	Purchase of safety item is required for all shaded boxes (✔ = item purchased)
General Indoor Safety *(continued)*		
14. Ensure that electric cords are not frayed or overloaded. Place out of a child's reach.		
15. Install "shock stops" (plastic outlet plugs) or outlet covers on all electric outlets.		☐ **Safety item — plastic outlet plugs**
16. To prevent falls, always keep one hand on the infant while he or she is on a high surface such as a changing table.		
17. Position healthy full-term infants on their back or side to sleep. *Do not place infants on their stomach to sleep.*		
18. The crib is safe. ■ The crib mattress fits snugly with no more than 2 fingers' breadth between the mattress and crib railing. ■ The distance between crib slats is less than 2⅜ inches (so the infant's head won't get caught).		
19. Check the strength of stairs, railings, porches, and balconies.		
20. Light hallways and stairways to prevent falls.		
21. Use toddler gates at the top and bottom of stairs. (Do not use accordion-type gates with wide spaces at the top. They can entrap a child's head and cause strangulation.)		☐ **Safety item — toddler gates (NOT accordion-type)**
22. Do not let your child use an infant walker.		
23. To prevent falls, place locks (available at hardware stores) on all windows. Put gates on the lower part of open windows.		☐ **Safety item — window locks, gates**
24. Store medicines and vitamins out of a child's reach and in child-resistant containers.		☐ **Safety item — child-resistant containers**
25. Store cleaning products out of a child's reach and sight. ■ Store and label all household poisons in their original containers in high locked cabinets (not under sinks). ■ Do not store chemicals or poisons in soda bottles. ■ Store cleaning products separately from food.		

	I follow this safety precaution (✔ = yes)	Purchase of safety item is required for all shaded boxes (✔ = item purchased)
General Indoor Safety *(continued)*		
26. Install safety latches or locks on cabinets that contain potentially **dangerous items and are within a child's reach.**		☐ **Safety item — safety latches or locks on cabinets**
27. Keep purses containing vitamins, medications, cigarettes, matches, jewelry, and calculators (which have easy-to-swallow button batteries) out of a child's reach.		
28. Install a lock or hook-and-eye latch on the door leading to the basement or garage to prevent children from entering those areas. Place a lock at the top of the door frame.		☐ **Safety item — latch on basement, garage doors**
29. Keep potentially harmful plants out of a child's reach. (Many plants are poisonous. Consult your poison control center.)		
30. Be sure that toy chests have lightweight lids, no lids, or safe-closing hinges.		
Kitchen Safety		
31. To minimize the risk of burns: ■ Keep hot liquids, foods, and cooking utensils out of a child's reach. ■ Place hot liquids and food away from the edge of the table. ■ Cook on the back burners when possible and turn pot handles toward the center of the stove. ■ Avoid using tablecloths and place mats that can be yanked off, spilling hot liquids or food. ■ Keep high chairs and stools away from the stove. ■ Do not keep snacks near the stove. ■ Teach young children the meaning of the word *hot*.		
32. Keep all foods and small items (including balloons) that can choke a child out of reach. Test toys for size with a toilet-paper roll (if it fits inside the roll, it can choke a small child).		
33. Keep knives and other sharp objects out of a child's reach.		
Bathroom Safety		
34. Bathe children in no more than 1 or 2 inches of water. Stay with infants and young children throughout the bath.		

	I follow this safety precaution (✔ = yes)	Purchase of safety item is required for all shaded boxes (✔ = item purchased)
Bathroom Safety *(continued)*		
35. Use skidproof mats or stickers in the bathtub.		☐ **Safety item — bath mats or stickers**
36. Adjust the maximum temperature of the water heater to 120° to 130°F (48.9° to 54.4°C) or medium heat (test with a thermometer).		
37. Keep electrical appliances (radios, hair dryers, space heaters, etc) out of the bathroom or unplugged, away from water, and out of a child's reach.		
Firearms		
38. If firearms are stored in the home, they must be locked and inaccessible to children. Store guns individually locked and unloaded, and store ammunition separately.		☐ **Safety item — trigger lock, lockboxes for firearms**
Outdoor Safety		
39. Playground equipment is assembled and anchored correctly according to manufacturer's instructions over a level, cushioned surface such as sand or wood chips.		
40. Your child knows the rules of safe bicycling. ■ Wear a protective helmet. ■ Use the correct size bicycle. ■ Ride on the right side of the road (*with* traffic). ■ Use hand signals and wear bright or reflective clothing.		☐ **Safety item — bicycle helmet**
41. Do not allow children to play with fireworks.		
42. Your child is properly protected while roller skating or skateboarding. ■ Child wears helmet and protective padding on knees and elbows. ■ Child skates only in rinks or parks that are free of traffic.		☐ **Safety item — helmet and protective padding**
43. Your child is properly protected while riding on sleds or snow disks. ■ Child sleds only in daylight and only in a safe, supervised area away from motor vehicles.		
44. Your child is properly protected while participating in contact sports. ■ Proper adult instruction and supervision are provided. ■ Teammates are of similar weight and size. ■ Appropriate safety equipment is used.		☐ **Safety item — safety equipment for contact sports**

	I follow this safety precaution (✔ = yes)	Purchase of safety item is required for all shaded boxes (✔ = item purchased)
Outdoor Safety *(continued)*		
45. To reduce the risk of animal bites: ■ Teach your child how to handle and care for a pet. ■ Teach your child never to try to separate fighting animals, even when a familiar pet is involved. ■ Teach your child to avoid unfamiliar animals.		
46. If you have a home swimming pool, be sure the pool is totally enclosed with fencing at least 5 feet high and that all gates are self-closing and self-latching. There should be no direct access (without a locked gate) from the home into the pool area. In addition ■ Children must *always* be supervised by an adult when swimming. Never allow a child to swim alone. ■ Change young children from swimsuits into street clothes and remove all toys from the pool area at the end of swim time. ■ All adults and older children should learn CPR. ■ Pools on nearby properties should be protected from use by unsupervised children.		☐ **Safety item — 5-foot fence around swimming pool with self-closing, self-latching gate**

Note: Much of the safety information presented in this course is based on the SAFEHOME program developed by the Massachusetts Department of Public Health as part of its Statewide Comprehensive Injury Prevention Program and the Children's Traffic Safety Program at Vanderbilt University in Nashville, Tenn. The SAFEHOME program was funded by the Federal Division of Maternal and Child Health. The Children's Traffic Safety Program was funded by the Department of Transportation and the Tennessee Governor's Highway Safety Program.

Module 2

Chapter ⬤3 The ABCs of CPR
Techniques of Infant and Child CPR and Relief of Choking

Case Scenario

You have been called to help as a child is pulled out of the water at the beach. The child is 3 years old and limp, with blue lips. As soon as you reach the child, you confirm that he is unresponsive and send a second rescuer to phone 911. You open the airway with a jaw thrust, and you look, listen, and feel for breathing. The child is not breathing. You pinch the child's nose, hold the airway open, and deliver 2 breaths. The chest rises with each breath. The child shows no response to the 2 breaths (no normal breathing, coughing, or movement).

What should you do next? What should you do until EMS personnel arrive?

Learning Objectives

After reading this chapter you should be able to

1. Describe and demonstrate 1-rescuer CPR for an infant and a child with and without a barrier device
2. Recognize signs of severe or complete choking
3. Describe and demonstrate how to clear the airway of a responsive infant or child with complete choking

CPR: The Second Link in the Chain of Survival for Infants and Children

The steps of CPR form the second link in the AHA pediatric Chain of Survival. The steps in CPR consist of the *assessments* and *skills* needed to support the airway, breathing, and circulation. CPR is performed in 3 basic steps known as the ABCs of CPR: **A**irway, **B**reathing, and **C**irculation. At each step you first must assess the victim and then provide the support the victim requires (use the *skill*).

CPR is designed to deliver oxygen to the blood and to move that oxygenated blood to the brain and other vital organs until medical treatment can restore normal heart action. Two primary CPR skills are rescue breathing or ventilation (blowing) and chest compressions (pumping).

If you find an *unresponsive* child, shout for help and then begin to provide CPR — begin to assess and support the **ABCs.** If someone else is with you or responds to your shout for help, send that person to **phone 911** or other emergency response number (the third link in the AHA pediatric Chain of Survival). If you are alone, perform CPR for about 1 minute before you phone 911.

Critical Concepts

Infant and Child CPR

- Check response
- If the child is unresponsive, shout for help.
- Begin CPR.

Check response by shouting or calling to the child. Gently tap the child. If the child does not respond, shout for help. Then begin CPR. If other rescuers are present, send one to phone 911 (or other emergency response number) as soon as you determine that the child is unresponsive.

Critical Concepts

Alteration in Chain of Survival Sequence for Infants and Children With Heart Disease

Some infants and children are at high risk for developing sudden cardiac arrest as a result of heart disease. If a child with known heart disease suddenly collapses, it may be more appropriate to use the sequence of actions in the adult Chain of Survival rather than the pediatric Chain of Survival. If your child has heart disease, ask your child's doctor or nurse whether you should use the pediatric Chain of Survival sequence (perform CPR for about 1 minute and then phone 911 or other emergency response number) or the adult Chain of Survival (phone 911 or other emergency response number and then perform CPR). The adult Chain of Survival is presented in Module 1 of this manual.

Heart disease is the most common cause of sudden cardiac arrest in adults, but it is a relatively uncommon cause of cardiac arrest in infants and children. The typical cause of cardiac arrest in infants and children is lack of oxygen supply to the heart muscle caused by a breathing problem, respiratory arrest, or shock. Breathing emergencies can occur as a result of choking, suffocation, airway disease, lung disease, submersion (near-drowning), or injuries involving the airway or brain. If an infant or child stops breathing, cardiac arrest follows in a very short time. If you immediately provide rescue breathing for a victim with a breathing emergency, you may prevent cardiac arrest.

The next section presents the basic approach to CPR for an infant or child. For the purposes of this course, the term *infant* refers to a child less than 1 year old; *child* refers to a child who is 1 to 8 years old. For a child older than 8 years, use the steps of CPR for adults. See Module 1 for more information about adult CPR.

1. **Check response: Check whether the victim is responsive** by shouting, "Are you OK?" and gently tapping the victim.

    - **If the victim is unresponsive, shout for help and begin CPR.** If anyone responds to your shout, tell the responder to phone 911 (or other emergency response number). This activates the EMS system and ensures that professional help is on the way.

    - **If you are alone** and find an unresponsive infant or child, **begin CPR** and provide approximately 1 minute of CPR and then call 911.

    - Kneel at the victim's side near his head. The victim should be on his back on a firm surface, such as a table or the floor. If necessary, carefully turn the victim onto his back. Support the head and neck as you turn the victim. If you suspect the victim is injured, turn the head and neck and body as a unit.

2. **Airway: Open the airway.**

    - *Head tilt–chin lift:* Tilt the head back by lifting the chin gently with one hand while pushing down on the forehead with the other hand **(see Figure 3)**. When lifting the chin, place your fingers on the bony part of the chin and avoid compressing on the soft tissues of the neck or under the chin. Lifting the chin moves the tongue away from the back of the throat and prevents obstruction of the airway by the tongue. It creates an open airway.

    - *Jaw thrust:* If trauma to the head or neck is suspected, do not tilt the head or neck. Instead use the jaw-thrust technique to open the airway. Lift on the angles of the jaw. This moves the jaw and tongue forward and opens the airway without bending the neck **(see Figure 4)**.

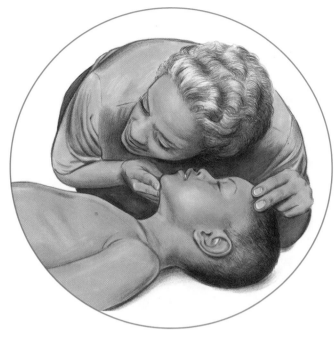

FIGURE 3.
Head tilt–chin lift. Open the airway with head tilt–chin lift by lifting the chin while pushing gently down on the forehead.

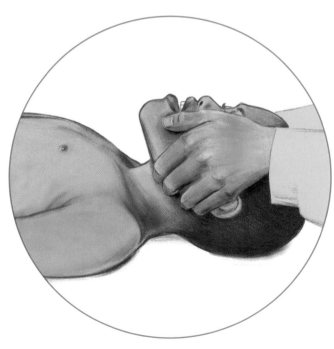

FIGURE 4.
Jaw thrust. Lift the angles of the jaw. This moves the jaw and the tongue forward and opens the airway without bending the neck.

3. **Breathing: Hold the airway open and look, listen, and feel to determine if the victim is breathing normally (see Figure 3). If the victim is not breathing normally, you will provide rescue breaths.**

To check for normal breathing, *look, listen,* and *feel* for the victim's breathing.

   a. Place your ear next to the victim's mouth and nose, turning your head to look at the chest.
   b. **Look** for the chest to rise. **Listen** and **feel** for air movement on your cheek.

If the victim is not breathing normally, give rescue breaths (see Figures 5 and 6).

To perform rescue breathing in an infant (see Figure 5), do the following:

   a. Cover the infant's mouth and nose with your mouth. If your mouth is too small to cover the infant's nose and mouth, cover the infant's nose with your mouth and deliver the rescue breaths through the infant's nose. You may need to hold the infant's mouth closed to prevent air from escaping through the mouth.
   b. Continue to tilt the head and lift the chin or perform jaw thrust.
   c. Give 2 slow breaths (1 to 1½ seconds for each breath).
   d. Be sure the infant's chest rises each time you give a rescue breath. The chest will rise if you are delivering enough air into the infant's lungs. Deliver just enough air to cause the infant's chest to rise. If the chest does not rise, reopen the airway and reattempt ventilation.
   e. If a barrier device suitable for infants is available for CPR, use the barrier device to provide rescue breathing (see "Barrier Devices and Masks" later in this chapter).

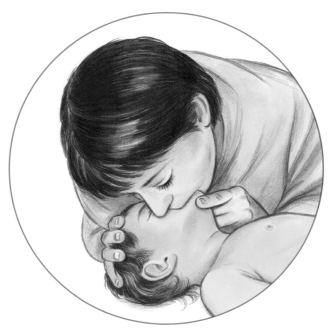

FIGURE 5.
Mouth-to-nose-and-mouth rescue breathing for an infant. The rescuer places her mouth over the infant's nose and mouth. If the rescuer cannot cover both the nose and mouth, she may cover the infant's nose alone to provide rescue breathing.

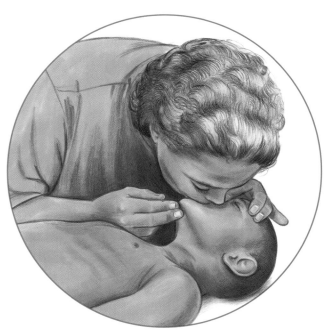

FIGURE 6A.
Mouth-to-mouth rescue breathing for a child. While keeping the child's airway open, the rescuer covers the child's mouth with her mouth and pinches the child's nose closed.

To perform rescue breathing in a child (see Figure 6A and B), do the following:

a. Cover the child's mouth with your mouth while pinching the child's nose closed.

b. Continue to hold the airway open by using a head tilt–chin lift or a jaw thrust.

c. Give 2 slow breaths (1 to 1½ seconds for each breath).

d. Be sure the child's chest rises each time you give a rescue breath. The chest will rise if you are delivering enough air into the child's lungs. If the chest does not rise, reopen the airway and reattempt ventilation.

e. If a barrier device is available for CPR, use the barrier device **(see Figure 6B)** to provide rescue breathing (see "Barrier and Mask Devices" later in this chapter).

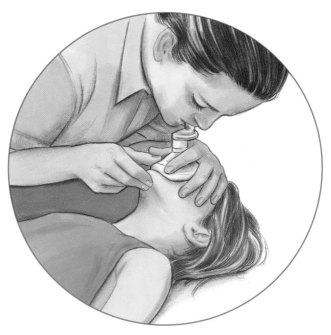

FIGURE 6B.
Rescue breathing with a barrier device. The rescuer must hold the barrier device tightly against the child's face while holding the airway open.

Foundation Facts

Facts About Respiratory Arrest and Rescue Breathing

Respiratory arrest is present when the infant or child stops breathing or breathes so slowly, shallowly, or irregularly that delivery of oxygen to the heart and brain is severely reduced. Remember, when breathing stops, oxygen delivery to the heart and brain soon stops. If oxygen delivery is not restored quickly, the heart and brain may be damaged. Mouth-to-mouth breathing is the fastest way to deliver oxygen to the victim's lungs and blood, and it may prevent development of cardiac arrest.

When providing rescue breathing, check to see that the victim's chest rises with each breath you give. This is the only way you can tell that you are giving good rescue breaths.

Deliver breaths slowly, using just enough volume to cause the victim's chest to rise. Take 1 to 1½ seconds to deliver each breath. Do not give rapid, large, forceful breaths, because you will blow air into the esophagus and stomach instead of the lungs. Air in the stomach can cause vomiting, which complicates CPR in many ways. *Remember, your lungs hold much more air than those of an infant or child. It is not necessary to blow a "full" breath for rescue breathing. You should blow just until you make the chest rise.*

After you provide 2 rescue breaths, check for signs of circulation. If you observe signs of circulation (normal breathing, coughing, or movement in response to the breaths), cardiac arrest is not present. Respiratory arrest may still be present, however. Be prepared to provide rescue breathing (1 breath every 3 seconds) if respiratory arrest is present.

When you look, listen, and feel for breathing and find that the victim is breathing, do not provide 2 rescue breaths. Observe the victim to be sure that breathing continues. If breathing continues, place the victim in the recovery position to keep the airway open **(see Figure 8).**

4. **Circulation**

   a. **Assess or check for signs of circulation in response to the 2 rescue breaths.** The victim has no signs of circulation if there is no response (no normal breathing, coughing, or movement) to the 2 breaths.

   b. Do not take more than 10 seconds to check for signs of circulation.

   c. **If you are not sure there are signs of circulation, begin chest compressions (see Figure 7A and B).**

   d. *Note:* If the victim has signs of circulation, chest compressions are *not* required. If the victim is not breathing normally but signs of circulation *are* present, the victim is in respiratory arrest. Continue rescue breathing (**1** breath every **3** seconds).

To provide chest compressions for an infant:

   a. Imagine a line drawn between the infant's nipples.

   b. Place 2 or 3 fingers of one hand on the infant's breastbone (sternum) about 1 finger's width below the imaginary line **(see Figure 7A).** Maintain head tilt with your other hand.

   c. Do not press over the very bottom of the breastbone (the xiphoid).

   d. To provide compressions, press the infant's chest downward about *one third to one half the depth* of the chest. Provide compressions at a rate of at least 100 compressions per minute.

Critical Concepts

Check for Signs of Circulation

Blood must circulate to deliver oxygen to the brain, heart, and other vital organs. If you can identify signs of normal breathing, coughing, or movement, the victim's heart is beating adequately to supply blood to the body, and chest compressions are unnecessary. If there is no response, the victim has no signs of circulation, and you must begin chest compressions to provide circulation to the body.

e. Release your pressure completely to allow the chest to expand after each compression, but do not move your fingers off the infant's chest.

f. Give **1** breath after every **5** compressions.

To provide chest compressions for a child:

a. Find the middle of the breastbone. Place the heel of one hand on the lower half of the breastbone but not over the very bottom of the sternum (the xiphoid) **(see Figure 7B).**

b. Maintain head tilt with your other hand (this will keep the airway open and facilitate the delivery of rescue breaths when needed).

c. Do not press over the very bottom of the sternum (the xiphoid).

d. To provide compressions, press the child's chest downward about *one third to one half the depth* of the chest. Provide compressions at a rate of approximately 100 compressions per minute.

e. Release your pressure completely to allow the chest to expand after each compression, but do not remove your hand from the child's chest.

f. Give **1** breath after every **5** compressions.

5. **"Pump and blow"*: Provide cycles of 5 chest compressions and 1 rescue breath.**

a. Continue CPR with 5 chest compressions ("pump") and 1 slow breath ("blow").

b. After providing CPR for approximately 1 minute (about 20 rescue breaths or 20 cycles of 5 compressions and 1 breath; these will actually take a little longer than 1 minute), check for signs of circulation (normal breathing, coughing, or movement).

c. If no signs of circulation are present and no one has phoned for help, leave the victim and **phone 911.** If the child is small and uninjured, you may carry him or her to the telephone to activate the EMS system. After you answer all of the dispatcher's questions, resume CPR.

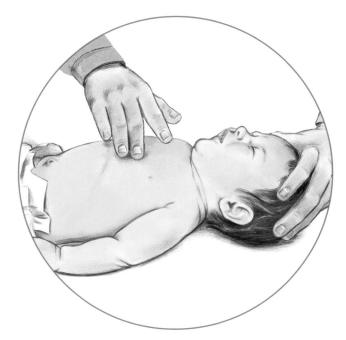

FIGURE 7A.
Two-fingered compressions for infants.

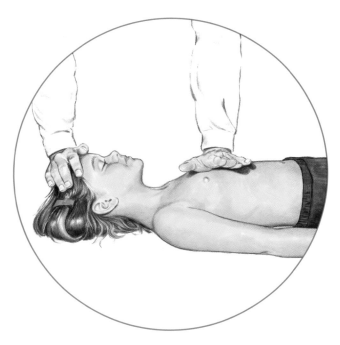

FIGURE 7B.
Chest compressions for children.

*Thanks to Allan Braslow, PhD, for coining the term *pump and blow* to describe chest compressions and rescue breathing.

d. Continue to provide chest compressions and rescue breathing (5 compressions and 1 rescue breath). Check for signs of circulation every few minutes. If signs of circulation return (the infant or child begins to breathe, cough, or move), stop chest compressions and continue rescue breathing if needed (1 breath every 3 seconds).

FYI...

Difference Between Compression Rate and Number of Compressions Actually Delivered per Minute

During infant CPR you compress the sternum at *a rate of at least 100 compressions per minute.* This corresponds to a rate that is slightly less than 2 compressions per second, so it will take only a few seconds to perform each set of 5 compressions. The compression *rate* refers to the *speed* of compressions, not to the actual number of compressions delivered per minute. Note that if you provide a compression *rate* of at least 100 compressions per minute, you will actually provide fewer than 100 compressions each minute because you will pause to provide ventilation (a slow breath) after every fifth compression. The actual number of compressions delivered per minute will vary from rescuer to rescuer and will be influenced by the compression rate and the speed with which you can position the head, open the airway, and deliver the rescue breath.

FYI...

Two-Rescuer CPR

CPR can also be performed by 2 rescuers. One rescuer assesses the victim and provides rescue breathing. The other (second) rescuer gives chest compressions. With 2 rescuers you use the same ratio of chest compressions and rescue breaths as used in 1-rescuer CPR: 5 compressions and 1 ventilation in each cycle.

Two-rescuer CPR may be taught as a module of the Heartsaver CPR Course. Your instructor will provide a 2-rescuer CPR Performance Criteria sheet if needed in your course.

Barrier Devices and Masks

Mouth-to-mouth rescue breathing may be life-saving for victims and is safe for rescuers. When you perform CPR you have almost no chance of becoming infected with viruses such as HIV (the virus that causes AIDS) or any of the hepatitis viruses. To date no human has ever contracted HIV or hepatitis through mouth-to-mouth contact during CPR.

Some potential rescuers may hesitate to perform mouth-to-mouth rescue breathing because of concerns about infectious diseases. It is important to remember that approximately 70% of CPR is performed in the home or for a loved one or friend.

The AHA recommends the use of barrier devices to encourage bystanders to start CPR if they are concerned about mouth-to-mouth contact with the victim. The Occupational Safety and Health Administration recommends that barrier devices be available in the workplace and that employees who perform CPR in the workplace (for example, security guards and shopping mall employees) use barrier devices to prevent the spread of infection. However, a barrier device is not *required* to provide CPR.

Do *not* withhold rescue breathing from a victim of cardiac or respiratory arrest just because a barrier device is not immediately available. If you waste time trying to locate a device and remember how to use it, you may reduce the victim's chance of survival.

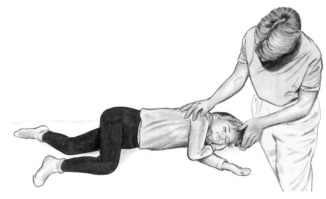

FIGURE 8.
The recovery position.

Regardless of whether a barrier device is available, the key actions of the rescuer remain the same: (1) Open the airway using the head tilt–chin lift maneuver (or jaw thrust if the victim has head or neck injuries), and (2) provide rescue breaths over 1 to 1½ seconds for each breath. When a barrier device is used, the rescuer positions the face shield or mask securely over the victim's mouth, ensuring an adequate air seal. *Rescue breathing should be delivered through the barrier device with a force sufficient to make the chest rise.*

There are 2 types of barrier devices, face shields and face masks. In the Heartsaver CPR Course for Infant and Child you will learn about the barrier device that you will use during actual rescue breathing and CPR. Correct use requires practice. Practice on a manikin several times. The most critical step in using a face shield or mask is achieving a good seal around the mouth and nose because this prevents leakage of air during rescue breathing.

Face Shields

Face shields are clear plastic or silicon sheets that you place over the victim's face to keep your mouth from directly touching the victim. All face shields have an opening or tube in the center of the plastic sheet. This allows your rescue breaths to enter the victim's mouth. Face shields are small, flexible, and portable. A folded shield will fit easily in a packet on a key ring. If you keep the packet on your key ring, it is much more likely to be available when you need it.

Face Masks

Face masks are made of firmer plastic than face shields **(see Figure 9).** These rigid devices fit over both the mouth and nose. Face masks contain a 1-way valve to prevent movement of germs between the victim and rescuer. Although face masks are easier to use than shields, they are bulkier, more expensive, and inconvenient to carry around, which means they are less likely to be available if you must perform CPR unexpectedly.

Using a Face Mask

Position yourself at the side of the victim's head in a location that will enable you to perform both rescue breathing and chest compressions, and do the following:

- Place the mask on the victim's face, using the bridge of the nose as a guide for correct position.
- Seal the mask by placing the index and thumb of your hand closest to the top of the victim's head along the border of the mask and placing the thumb of your other hand along the lower margin of the mask.
- Place the remaining fingers of your hand closest to the victim's feet along the bony margin of the jaw and lift the jaw while performing a head tilt **(see Figure 6B).**
- Compress firmly and completely around the outside margin of the mask to provide a tight seal.
- Provide slow rescue breaths. Be sure that the chest rises with each breath.

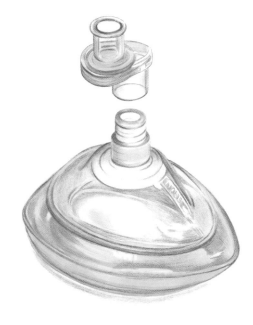

FIGURE 9.
Face masks are rigid devices that fit over the mouth and nose of the victim. They contain a 1-way valve to prevent movement of germs between the victim and rescuer.

Choking: Foreign-Body Airway Obstruction

Choking is an alarming and dramatic emergency. The desperate efforts of the choking infant or child to clear his or her airway heighten the emotional drama and increase the pressure on the rescuer to take the correct action.

How to Recognize Severe or Complete Choking in a Responsive Infant or Child

Choking should be suspected any time an infant or child *suddenly* chokes and begins to cough, gag, or have high-pitched, noisy breathing. An older child may also use the universal sign of choking, clutching the neck with one or both hands **(see Figure 10).**

Foreign objects may *partially* block the airway but still allow adequate air movement. Victims with partial obstruction of the airway remain responsive, can cough forcefully (produce a loud cough), and can usually speak or cry. Breath sounds may be noisy, and you may hear wheezing between coughs. *If the airway is only partially obstructed, do **not** attempt to relieve the obstruction.* If you have any concern about the child's breathing, **phone 911** to transport the child to the Emergency Department.

Victims with *severe or complete* airway obstruction will not be able to move enough air to make much sound (they cannot speak or cough forcefully). They may make very soft, high-pitched, or wheezing sounds when they try to breathe. When severe or complete airway obstruction is present, you must act quickly to relieve the obstruction. Other signs of complete obstruction include indications that the child is struggling to breathe (the ribs and chest sink in, or retract, when the infant or child tries to breathe in) and blueness of the lips and skin.

Foundation Facts

Causes of Airway Obstruction in Infants and Children

There are 3 common ways an infant's or child's airway may become obstructed. Each is treated differently.

1. **Foreign body.** A foreign body (for example, food, a toy, or a piece of a balloon) may become lodged in the air passage and produce severe or complete airway obstruction. This obstruction prevents the infant or child from breathing effectively. If you remove the foreign body immediately, the infant or child can resume normal breathing. To remove the object, deliver back blows and chest thrusts to the infant and abdominal thrusts to the child (Heimlich maneuver). Repeat these maneuvers until the object is dislodged or the infant becomes unresponsive. If the victim becomes unresponsive, attempt CPR.

2. **Relaxed tongue.** In an unresponsive victim (for example, following a head injury), the tongue may fall back against the throat, blocking the airway. Use either the head tilt–chin lift maneuver or the jaw-thrust maneuver (for victims with possible head or neck injury) to lift the tongue away from the back of the throat. No back blows, chest thrusts, or abdominal thrusts are needed.

3. **Swollen air passages.** This condition is a *medical* problem rather than one caused by a foreign body. Swelling of the airways can result from conditions such as asthma, infection (for example, croup), or allergy. Positioning of the head or neck, back blows, chest thrusts, and the Heimlich maneuver will ***not*** eliminate this form of airway obstruction. If the victim stops breathing, give rescue breaths slowly, while maintaining a tight mouth-to-mouth seal, making sure the chest rises with each breath.

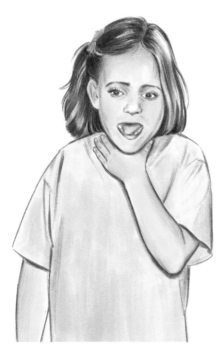

FIGURE 10.
Universal choking sign in a child.

The following signs are *red flags,* or major warning signs, of severe or complete airway obstruction in a responsive infant or child. If you see any of the following signs, act immediately to relieve the obstruction:

- Universal sign of choking (clutching the neck with one or both hands; **see Figure 10).** Ask, "Are you choking?" (The child may nod.)
- Inability to speak, cough forcefully, or cry (the child may have ineffective, weak coughs). Ask, "Can you speak?" (The child will shake her head "NO").
- Weak, ineffective coughs
- High-pitched sounds or no sounds while breathing in.
- Bluish lips or skin.

First Aid for Severe or Complete Choking

This section describes the **actions you perform to dislodge a foreign object** that is causing severe or complete obstruction of the airway in a responsive infant or child. Perform these actions when the responsive infant or child has signs of

severe or complete airway obstruction and you suspect the obstruction is caused by a foreign object (for example, if a child playing with a small toy suddenly starts to cough forcefully and then cannot talk or make other sounds). **Do *not* follow these steps** if the cause of obstruction is illness (for example, the infant or child has been ill with asthma or has a croupy or hoarse cough).

Relief of Complete Foreign-Body Airway Obstruction in a Responsive Infant

1. Position the infant face down and head down while you support the infant's jaw and head with your hand. Often you will need to sit or kneel, resting the arm holding the infant's torso on your lap or thigh.
2. Deliver up to **5** back blows with the heel of your free hand **(see Figure 11A).** If the object is expelled and the infant begins to breathe after fewer than 5 back blows, discontinue the back blows.
3. If the obstruction is not expelled after 5 back blows, turn the infant onto his or her back while supporting the head and deliver up to **5** chest thrusts using 2 to 3 fingers positioned over the breastbone (sternum) in the same position used for chest compression during CPR **(see Figure 11B).** Deliver each thrust with the intention of dislodging the object by deliberately compressing the chest. Stop chest compressions if the object is dislodged.
4. Alternate performing **5** back blows and **5** chest compressions until the object is dislodged or the infant becomes unresponsive.

Relief of Complete Foreign-Body Airway Obstruction in a Responsive Child

In children the **Heimlich maneuver** (abdominal thrusts) is used to relieve complete obstruction of the airway caused by a foreign object. The Heimlich maneuver quickly forces air from the victim's lungs, similar to a cough. The rapid air movement expels the blocking object like a cork from a bottle.

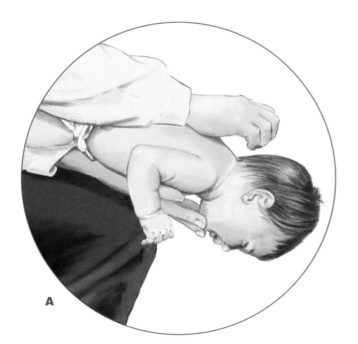
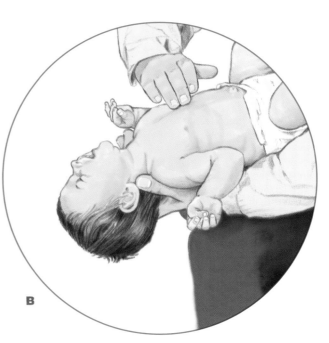

FIGURE 11.
Relief of choking in the responsive infant. **A.** Back blows. **B.** Chest thrusts.

1. Tell the child you are going to help him or her. Stand behind the child and wrap your arms around the child so that your fists are in front of the child **(see Figure 12).**
2. Make a fist with one hand.
3. Place the thumb side of the fist on the child's abdomen slightly above the navel and below the breastbone.
4. Grasp the fist with the other hand and provide quick upward thrusts into the child's abdomen.
5. Give sets of 5 abdominal thrusts and watch to see if the object is expelled.
6. Repeat sets of abdominal thrusts until the object is expelled or the child becomes unresponsive.

If complete airway obstruction is *not* relieved, the infant or child will become unresponsive and may turn blue. The infant or child may also stop breathing. When this happens, the brain and heart do not have enough oxygen-rich blood to function well. When the child becomes unresponsive, shout for help and begin CPR. Open the airway widely and look for the object. If you see it, remove it. If the child is not breathing,

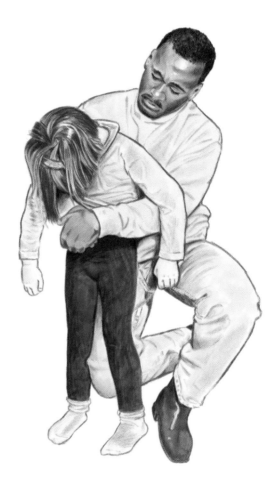

FIGURE 12.
Relief of choking in the responsive child. Abdominal thrusts (Heimlich maneuver).

give 2 rescue breaths. If the child has no signs of circulation after you deliver 2 rescue breaths, begin chest compressions. The chest compressions may dislodge the object. If these interventions are not effective after about 1 minute, **phone 911** unless another rescuer has already done so.

Keeping Your Skills Sharp: CPR Practice

Review the steps and skills of rescuer CPR regularly (several times every year). Reread this manual. Use practice videos and CPR prompt devices to enhance your practice. Renew your CPR skills with an instructor at least every 2 years by taking an AHA renewal course. **Never rehearse or practice CPR skills on another person.** Chest compressions can be lifesaving during CPR, but they can injure a responsive, healthy person.

The Heartsaver CPR Course for Infant and Child teaches you how to prevent death caused by SIDS and injury. It also teaches you how to recognize the signs of breathing emergencies (including choking) and respiratory and cardiac arrest, the steps of infant and child CPR, and how to treat complete foreign-body airway obstruction. The Heartsaver CPR adult course provides information about CPR for adults and treatment of choking in adults.

Summary

Everyone who cares for infants and children should know how to prevent arrest and injuries, how to recognize cardiac and breathing emergencies, and how to provide CPR and relieve choking. This chapter has presented the ABCs of CPR (airway, breathing, and circulation) and the assessment and skills steps of CPR.

Problems with the **airway** are common. Everyone should know how to

- Open the airway of an unresponsive victim
- Relieve choking in a responsive infant or child

Problems with **breathing** occur in cases of

- Respiratory and cardiac arrest
- Submersion (near-drowning) injury
- Head trauma
- Poisoning
- Asthma, infection of the airway, or allergic reaction

To manage severe breathing problems, you need to know how to open the airway and give rescue breaths. You must deliver rescue breaths slowly and gently to make the chest rise.

Problems with **circulation** occur during cardiac arrest. *Chest compressions* are needed if the victim has no signs of circulation. An infant or child who is unresponsive, is not breathing, and has no response to 2 rescue breaths is probably in **cardiac arrest** *and requires a combination of rescue breathing and chest compressions.* The combination of rescue breathing and chest compressions will deliver oxygenated blood to the brain, heart, and other vital organs. The actions of pumping (chest compressions) are simple and easy to learn.

Learning Checklist

Take a moment to review the key information you have learned in this chapter before evaluating your knowledge.

✔ When you encounter an infant or child in distress, perform the following actions first:

1. Determine responsiveness. If the victim is unresponsive, shout for help.
2. Open the airway and assess breathing.
3. If the victim is not breathing, give 2 slow breaths, making sure the chest rises.

4. Check for signs of circulation (breathing, coughing, or movement) in response to the 2 breaths. If there are no signs of circulation, start chest compressions.

5. If you are alone, give CPR for 1 minute and then phone 911.

✔ Open the airway using the head tilt–chin lift maneuver. Use the jaw-thrust maneuver to open the airway if you suspect that the head or neck is injured. Then look, listen, and feel for breathing.

1. Turn your head to observe the chest: **Look for the chest to rise.**

2. Place your ear next to the victim's mouth and nose: **Listen for breathing.**

3. **Feel for air movement** on your cheek.

✔ If the victim is not breathing normally, deliver 2 rescue breaths, making the chest rise with each breath. After you deliver 2 rescue breaths, check for signs of circulation. If there are no signs of circulation (no breathing, coughing, or movement), begin chest compressions.

- In infants compress the breastbone or sternum about 1 finger's width below the nipple line. In children compress the lower half of the child's breastbone or sternum.
- Do not press the very bottom of the sternum (the xiphoid).
- In infants and children compress one third to one half the depth of the chest.
- Provide compressions at a rate of *at least* 100 compressions per minute for the infant and approximately 100 compressions per minute for the child.
- After every 5 compressions provide 1 rescue breath (ventilation).

✔ During CPR for infants and children the ratio of compressions to ventilations (breaths) is 5 to 1.

✔ After giving CPR for 1 minute, recheck the victim for signs of circulation and phone 911 (or other emergency response number) if this has not been done by another rescuer.

✔ Place any victim who is unresponsive but breathing in the recovery position unless you suspect that the victim's neck is injured.

✔ The red flags or major warning signs of a severe or complete foreign-body airway obstruction are

- Universal sign of choking (clutching the neck with 1 or 2 hands)
- Inability to make a sound (victim cannot speak, cough forcefully, or cry)
- Ability to make only very high-pitched or wheezing sounds while inhaling
- Increased difficulty breathing
- Bluish lips, tongue, and skin (cyanosis)

✔ In responsive infants complete airway obstruction is relieved by alternating sets of 5 back blows with sets of 5 chest compressions until the object is expelled or the infant becomes unresponsive. If the infant becomes unresponsive, begin CPR.

✔ In responsive children complete airway obstruction is relieved by performing abdominal thrusts (the Heimlich maneuver). Place your fist just above the navel and well below the breastbone and then rapidly compress the abdomen. Repeat abdominal thrusts until the object is dislodged or the child becomes unresponsive. If the child becomes unresponsive, begin CPR.

Review Questions

1. **Your neighbor calls urgently for you because she is worried about her 2-year-old daughter, who suddenly became limp. Which of the following responses indicates the correct order of steps you should perform?**

   a. verify that the child is unresponsive, phone 911, check for signs of circulation, open the airway, give 2 breaths if needed

   b. open the airway, verify that the child is unresponsive, give 2 breaths if needed, check for signs of circulation, phone 911 if the child has no pulse

   c. verify that the child is unresponsive, tell your neighbor to phone 911, open the airway, check for breathing, give 2 breaths if needed, and check for signs of circulation

   d. verify that the child is unresponsive, give 2 breaths, check for signs of circulation, phone 911, begin chest compressions

2. **You are at the food court in a shopping mall, and a mother begins shouting that her child is choking and needs help. You run over to the table to find an infant who is about 10 months old. The infant is awake and apparently struggling to breathe. She looks alarmed but is not making a sound; she is not coughing or speaking. Her lips are dusky. You see a plate with pieces of hot dog on the table in front of the infant. The mother says the infant began coughing and gagging while eating the hot dog and then suddenly became silent. You tell the mother and the infant that you are going to try to help. What is your next action?**

   a. give 5 back blows followed by 5 chest compressions until the hot dog is expelled or the infant becomes unresponsive

   b. give up to 5 abdominal thrusts (the Heimlich maneuver) until the hot dog is expelled or the child becomes unresponsive

   c. attempt to provide rescue breathing

   d. open the airway and perform a blind finger sweep

3. **You are unsuccessful in dislodging the hot dog, and the infant becomes unresponsive. You send the mother to phone 911, and you lay the infant on the floor to begin CPR. You open the airway widely, and you see a piece of hot dog in the back of the infant's throat. You remove it, hold the airway open, and note that the infant is not breathing. What should you do next?**

   a. give 2 rapid, forceful breaths

   b. give 1 slow breath

   c. check for signs of circulation

   d. give 2 slow breaths, making the chest rise

4. **After you deliver rescue breaths, you check for signs of circulation. What signs of circulation should you look for?**

   a. the infant should breathe normally, cough, or move in response to the rescue breaths

   b. the infant should follow commands

   c. the infant should demonstrate the universal choking sign

   d. nothing; there are no reliable signs of circulation in the infant

5. **You observe no signs of circulation, and you prepare to perform chest compressions. Which of the following responses gives the correct compression rate and the ratio of compressions (pumping) to ventilations (blowing) for an infant?**

   a. give 15 compressions and 2 ventilations at a compression rate of 60 compressions per minute

   b. give 5 compressions and 1 ventilation at a compression rate of no more than 60 compressions per minute

   c. give 15 compressions and 2 ventilations at a compression rate of 100 compressions per minute

   d. give 5 compressions and 1 ventilation at a compression rate of at least 100 compressions per minute

6. **Where should you position your hand to perform chest compressions in this 10-month-old infant?**

   a. over a line drawn between the 2 nipples
   b. 1 finger's width below the nipple line
   c. 1 finger's width above the nipple line
   d. over the very bottom of the breastbone (sternum)

7. **What is the best sign that your rescue breaths are providing air to the victim's lungs?**

   a. the victim's color changes
   b. the victim's pulse is visible in the neck
   c. the victim's chest rises with each breath
   d. you need medical equipment to determine whether you are providing air to the lungs

8. **A child begins to cough forcefully and loudly while eating. You should immediately**

   a. give abdominal thrusts
   b. give several back blows followed by several chest thrusts until the object is expelled or the child becomes unresponsive
   c. phone 911 or other emergency response number
   d. be prepared to act if signs of severe or complete foreign-body airway obstruction develop

9. **You are walking down the hallway of an elementary school and are called to the bathroom, where a 6-year-old with a known seizure disorder is reportedly unresponsive. Which of the following indicates the most appropriate order of actions you should be prepared to take?**

   a. verify that the child is unresponsive and then ask someone to phone 911 while you open the airway to assess breathing
   b. begin rescue breathing, check for signs of circulation, determine the child's response to voice, and ask someone to phone 911
   c. ask someone to phone 911 and place the child in the recovery position
   d. perform abdominal thrusts (the Heimlich maneuver)

10. **You find that the child in the previous question does not respond to voice or stimulation, takes only an occasional shallow breath, and has bluish lips. What should be your next actions?**

    a. begin chest compressions and ventilations at a ratio of 5 to 1
    b. provide 2 rescue breaths and evaluate her response
    c. place her in the recovery position and wait for EMS personnel to arrive
    d. perform abdominal thrusts (the Heimlich maneuver)

How did you do?

1, c; **2,** a; **3,** d; **4,** a; **5,** d; **6,** b; **7,** c; **8,** d; **9,** a; **10,** b.

Module 2

Chapter **4** *The Human Dimension of CPR*

Case Scenario

You provided CPR for a young child at the beach while the father watched helplessly. The child was still blue and lifeless when the paramedics arrived. They continued CPR, placed the child on a monitor, inserted a breathing tube, started an intravenous line, and transported the child to the hospital while providing ongoing CPR. You later learned that the child was pronounced dead in the Emergency Department. For several nights you awaken from restless sleep with visions of the child's lifeless body. You recall each detail of the CPR that you provided, wondering what you did wrong. You are having more and more difficulty sleeping, and you have lost your appetite. You are having trouble concentrating at work.

What could explain your distress following this "failed" attempt at CPR? What should you do?

Learning Objectives

After taking this course you should be able to do the following:

1. State how often CPR restores a victim's heartbeat and breathing in an out-of-hospital setting.
2. Give 2 different definitions of "success" of lay rescuer resuscitation.
3. State the importance of debriefing after a resuscitation attempt.
4. Explain the role of the debriefing facilitator.
5. Know who to contact after you have attempted resuscitation.

The Human Dimension of CPR: How Often Will Lay Rescuer CPR Succeed?

Since 1973 more than 40 million people have learned CPR. Many public health experts consider CPR training to be the most successful public health initiative of modern times. Millions of people have learned how to take action to save the life of a fellow human being. Unfortunately your best efforts will not succeed most of the time. Only 10% to 15% of children who have a cardiac arrest at home or in a public location survive to leave the hospital. One reason survival is so low is that few bystanders provide CPR. If CPR is not started before EMS personnel arrive, the child has little hope of survival. Survival is much higher when the infant or child has only a respiratory arrest and receives prompt rescue breathing from bystanders. If you are prepared to recognize emergencies, provide CPR, and phone 911 when needed, you may make a great difference in the life of an infant or child.

Even if you begin CPR immediately and perform it perfectly, many infants and children who have a cardiac arrest outside the hospital will not survive. For this reason it is important to briefly discuss the range of emotional reactions you might experience after a resuscitation attempt. Your reactions may be particularly intense when your efforts appear to have failed.

Take Pride in Your Skills as a Heartsaver CPR Rescuer

You should be proud that you are learning CPR. We hope you never have to use these skills, but emergencies happen. Now you can be confident that you will be better prepared to do the right thing for the children in your family and your community. Your efforts will not always restore life. But your success is not measured by whether a victim of cardiac arrest lives or dies. *You succeed when you recognize the emergency and try to help by using the CPR skills you have learned in this course.* Simply by taking action, making an effort, and just trying to help you will be judged a success.

Stress Reactions of Rescuers and Witnesses After Resuscitation Attempts

A cardiac arrest is a dramatic and emotional event, especially if the victim is an infant or child. The emergency may involve disagreeable physical details, such as bleeding or vomiting. Any emergency can be emotionally draining, especially if you are closely involved with the victim. The emergency can produce strong emotional reactions in bystanders, lay rescuers, and EMS professionals. Failed attempts at resuscitation can impose even more stress if the victim is someone you know. This stress can produce a variety of emotional reactions and physical symptoms that may last long after the original emergency. These reactions are common and normal.

It is **common** for a person to experience emotional aftershocks after an unpleasant event. Usually such stress reactions occur immediately after or within the first few hours after the event. Sometimes the emotional response may occur later.

Psychologists working with professional emergency personnel have learned that rescuers experience grief, anxiety, anger, and sometimes guilt. Typical physical reactions include difficulty sleeping, fatigue, irritability, changes in eating habits, and confusion. Many people say they are unable to stop thinking about the event.

Remember that these reactions are **common** and **normal.** They do not mean that you are "disturbed" or "weak." Strong reactions simply indicate that this particular event had a powerful impact on you. With the understanding and support of loved ones, these stress reactions usually pass quickly.

Techniques to Prevent and Reduce Stress in Rescuers, Families, and Witnesses

Psychologists have learned that the most successful way to reduce stress after rescue efforts is simple: *Talk about it.* Sit down with other people who witnessed the event and talk it over. EMS personnel are encouraged to offer emotional support to lay rescuers and bystanders. More formal discussions should include not only lay rescuers but also professional responders.

In these discussions you will be encouraged to describe what happened. Do not be frightened about "reliving" the event. Although such a fear is natural, talking about the event is a healthy way to deal with and overcome your fear. Describe the thoughts and feelings you experienced during the rescue effort. Describe how you feel now. Be patient with yourself. Understand that most reactions will diminish within a few days. Sharing your thoughts and feelings with your family, fellow rescuers, EMS personnel, friends, or clergy will can prevent or reduce stress reactions and help with your recovery.

In some communities EMS leaders may establish plans for more formal discussions or debriefings after resuscitations. Such sessions are called **"critical incident stress debriefings,"** or critical event debriefings.

Teams of specially trained persons are available to organize and conduct these debriefings. Such persons are usually associated with EMS services, employee assistance programs, community mental health centers, or public school systems. Other sources of psychological and emotional support can be local clergy, police chaplains, fire service chaplains, or hospital and Emergency Department social workers.

A critical event debriefing is a confidential group process. The facilitator leads and encourages persons involved in a stressful situation to express their thoughts and feelings about the event. You do not have to talk during the briefing, but if you do, what you say may help you and reassure others. The discussions are confidential and are not shared outside the group without permission. Rescuers and witnesses to an event can express and discuss feelings they experienced during and after a resuscitation attempt. These feelings may include guilt, anxiety, anger, or failure, especially if the resuscitation attempt was unsuccessful. Ideally the rescuers who were most involved in the resuscitation should be present for the debriefing. In some EMS programs EMS personnel visit the lay rescuers who were involved in the resuscitation effort.

Psychological Barriers to Action

This course is preparing you to respond appropriately to a future emergency. Although you are preparing yourself by taking this course, chances are that you will never have to use your skills. Most laypersons have never been close to a victim of cardiac arrest and have seen CPR performed only on television or in the movies.

Reality is quite different. During your Heartsaver CPR Course and while reading this handbook, you may have had some troubling thoughts.

Here are some common concerns lay rescuers express about responding to sudden emergencies. *Will I really have what it takes to respond to a true emergency?* Any emergency involving a family member, loved one, or neighbor will produce strong emotional reactions. Parents, for example, sometimes feel paralyzed during the first few moments of an emergency in which their child is a victim. *Will I be able to take action? Will I remember the steps of CPR?* These are common concerns.

What about the unpleasant and disagreeable aspects of doing CPR? *Would I be able to perform mouth-to-mouth rescue breathing on a stranger? What if the victim is bleeding from facial injuries that occurred when he or she collapsed? What if the victim vomits during CPR? Would this pose a risk of disease for a rescuer without a CPR barrier device?*

Often friends, relatives, or coworkers will be present at the emergency. If you respond and take action, these people will often be willing to help, but they may look to you for instruction. It may be difficult to act decisively during such a rare and challenging event.

It is well known that these psychological barriers hinder a quick emergency response, especially by ordinary citizens who seldom face such an event. There are no easy solutions to help overcome these psychological barriers. Your instructor will encourage you to anticipate many of the scenes described above. The practice scenarios will include role playing and rehearsals. Think through how you would like to respond if confronted with an emergency. Mental practice, even without hands-on practice, is a good technique for improving future performance.

The AHA Emergency Cardiovascular Care Committee encourages you to practice the skills you have learned and review the information in this manual every few months. The required renewal interval for CPR classes is **every 2 years.** These home practice sessions and instructor-supervised renewal sessions will strengthen your skills, build your confidence, and increase the probability of a smooth and effective resuscitative effort. Remember your goal: to help someone in need and perhaps to save the life of an infant or child.

Legal Aspects of CPR

The AHA has supported community CPR training for more than 3 decades. Lay CPR rescuers have helped save thousands of lives.

Lay rescuers can perform emergency CPR without fear of legal action. Chest compressions and rescue breathing require direct physical contact between rescuer and victim, 2 people who may be strangers. Too often the arrest victim dies. In the United States people may take legal action when they perceive damage or think that one person has harmed another even if the harm was unintentional. Despite this litigious environment, CPR remains widely used and remarkably free of legal issues and lawsuits. Although attorneys have included rescuers who performed CPR in lawsuits, no **"Good Samaritan"** has ever been found guilty of doing harm while performing CPR.

All 50 states have Good Samaritan laws that grant immunity to anyone who attempts CPR in an honest, "good faith" effort to save a life. A person is considered a Good Samaritan if

- He or she is genuinely trying to help.
- The help is reasonable (the rescuer cannot engage in gross misconduct).
- The rescue effort is voluntary (the rescuer is not paid for the resuscitative effort).

Under most Good Samaritan laws laypersons are protected if they perform CPR even if they have had no formal training.

Summary

Be proud of yourself for taking the Heartsaver CPR Course. Be proud of your new skills as a lay rescuer who can provide assistance and activate the EMS system to save a life.

Despite all the excitement about having the knowledge and skills to provide CPR, there are limits to what your efforts will achieve. This explains the emphasis on prevention of SIDS and injury in this course. Unfortunately, competent CPR will not always save a life. What is important is taking action and trying to help another human being. Some people must overcome psychological barriers to action if asked to respond to a dramatic emergency such as cardiac arrest. Taking the Heartsaver CPR Course will reduce many of these barriers. Feel free to express your concerns openly during the course and small-group sessions.

All EMS programs are encouraged to acknowledge the mental and emotional challenge of rescue efforts. You will have support from these programs if you ever participate in a resuscitation attempt. You may not know for several days whether the victim lives or dies. If the person you tried to resuscitate does not live, take comfort in knowing that in taking action, you did your best.

Learning Checklist

✔ CPR attempts are often unsuccessful. Your efforts will not always succeed.

✔ The most successful way to reduce stress after rescue efforts is to talk about it.

✔ Formal discussions or debriefings after resuscitations are called "critical incident stress debriefings."

✔ Some people must overcome barriers to action if asked to respond to a cardiac arrest.

✔ There has never been a lawsuit in which a lay rescuer was found guilty of doing harm in attempting CPR on a victim of cardiac arrest.

✔ Your success will be measured by the fact that you tried.

Review Questions

1. **A friend who helped you perform CPR 2 days ago says she is experiencing fatigue, irritability, difficulty sleeping, guilt, loss of appetite, shortness of breath, anxiety, and depression. These are likely signs of**

   a. heart attack
   b. impending cardiac arrest
   c. stress response
   d. heart failure

2. **Your friend who is experiencing the symptoms described in Question 1 asks what she should do to address this problem. You suggest that she attend a group meeting led by a physician, social worker, or other professional in which she can express her feelings. What is the term for this type of meeting?**

   a. Critical incident stress debriefing
   b. Analysis
   c. Biofeedback
   d. Psychological ventilation

3. **An emergency physician approaches you after an unsuccessful resuscitation attempt to ask how he and his associates can help to reduce your stress after the event. What role might you suggest for the physician that would be helpful to you and other rescuers after a resuscitation attempt?**

   a. Facilitator of a debriefing process
   b. Observer of a debriefing process
   c. Passive participant
   d. No particular role

How did you do?

1, c; **2,** a; **3,** a.

Heartsaver CPR Course for Infant and Child

Infant 1-Rescuer CPR
Performance Criteria

American Heart Association®

Fighting Heart Disease and Stroke

Student Name_____ Date _____

Performance Guidelines	Performed
1. Establish unresponsiveness. If a bystander is available, send that person to phone 911 (or other emergency response number).	
2. Open the airway (head tilt–chin lift or, if trauma is suspected, jaw thrust). Check for normal breathing (look, listen, and feel).*	
3. Give 2 slow breaths (1 to 1½ seconds per breath), ensure adequate chest rise, and allow for exhalation between breaths.	
4. Check for signs of circulation (normal breathing, coughing, or movement in response to the 2 rescue breaths). If signs of circulation are present but normal breathing is absent, provide rescue breathing (1 breath every 3 seconds, about 20 breaths per minute).*	
5. If no signs of circulation are present, begin cycles of 5 chest compressions with the 2-finger technique (rate of at least 100 compressions per minute) followed by 1 slow breath.	
6. After about 1 minute of rescue support, check for signs of circulation.* If rescuer is alone, phone 911 (or other emergency response number). If no signs of circulation are present, continue 5:1 cycles of chest compressions and ventilations. If signs of circulation are present but normal breathing is absent, continue rescue breathing (1 breath every 3 seconds, about 20 per minute).*	

*If the victim is breathing or resumes normal breathing and no trauma is suspected, place in the recovery position.

Comments _____

_____

_____

Instructor _____

Circle one: Complete   Needs more practice

Heartsaver CPR Course for Infant and Child

Child 1-Rescuer CPR
Performance Criteria

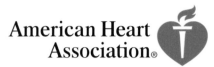

American Heart
Association®

Fighting Heart Disease and Stroke

Student Name _____ Date _____

Performance Guidelines	Performed
1. Establish unresponsiveness. If a bystander is available, send that person to phone 911 (or other emergency response number).	
2. Open the airway (head tilt–chin lift of, if trauma is suspected, jaw thrust). Check for normal breathing (look, listen, and feel).*	
3. Give 2 slow breaths (1 to 1½ seconds per breath), ensure adequate chest rise, and allow for exhalation between breaths.	
4. Check for signs of circulation (normal breathing, coughing, or movement in response to 2 breaths). If signs of circulation are present but normal breathing is absent, provide rescue breathing (1 breath every 3 seconds, about 20 breaths per minute).*	
5. If no signs of circulation are present, provide cycles of 5 chest compressions, typically with the 1-hand technique (rate of about 100 compressions per minute), followed by 1 slow breath.	
6. After about 1 minute of rescue support, check for signs of circulation.* If the rescuer is alone, phone 911 (or other emergency response number). If no signs of circulation are present, continue cycles of chest compressions and ventilations (5:1 ratio). If signs of circulation are present but normal breathing is absent, continue rescue breathing (1 breath every 3 seconds, about 20 breaths per minute).	

*If the victim is breathing or resumes normal breathing and no trauma is suspected, place in the recovery position.

Comments _____

_____

_____

Instructor _____

Circle one: Complete   Needs more practice

Infant or Child 2-Rescuer CPR (Optional) Performance Criteria

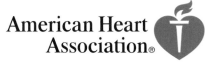

American Heart Association®

Fighting Heart Disease and Stroke

Student Name_____ Date _____

Performance Guidelines	Performed
1. Establish unresponsiveness. One rescuer should phone 911 (or other emergency response number).	
Rescuer 1	
2. Open the airway (head tilt–chin lift or, if trauma is suspected, jaw thrust). Check for normal breathing (look, listen, and feel).*	
3. If normal breathing is absent, give 2 slow breaths (1 to 1½ seconds per breath), ensure adequate chest rise, and allow for exhalation between breaths.	
4. Check for signs of circulation (normal breathing, coughing, or movement in response to 2 rescue breaths). If signs of circulation are present but normal breathing is absent, provide rescue breathing (1 breath every 3 seconds, about 20 breaths per minute).	
Rescuer 2	
5. If no signs of circulation are present, begin cycles of 5 chest compressions pausing briefly after each fifth compression to allow Rescuer 1 to provide 1 slow breath. Resume chest compressions at end of chest rise for breath.* • *Infant:* Use 2-finger technique at a rate of at least 100 compressions per minute. • *Child:* Use 1-hand technique at a rate of about 100 compressions per minute.	
6. After about 20 cycles of 5:1 compressions and ventilations (about 1 minute), Rescuer 1 provides 1 breath and rechecks for signs of circulation.* If no signs of circulation are present, continue 5:1 cycles of compressions and ventilations, beginning with chest compressions.	

*If the victim is breathing or resumes effective breathing, place in the recovery position.

Comments _____

_____

_____

Instructor _____

Circle one: Complete   Needs more practice

Heartsaver CPR Course for Infant and Child

Infant Foreign-Body Airway Obstruction in Responsive Victim
(and Responsive Victim Who Becomes Unresponsive)
Performance Criteria

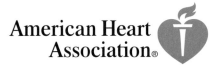

Fighting Heart Disease and Stroke

Student Name _____ Date _____

Performance Guidelines	Performed
1. Check for serious breathing difficulty, ineffective cough, and weak or absent cry). If severe or complete airway obstruction is present, proceed.	
2. Support the infant on rescuer's knee or lap and give 5 back blows with heel of hand followed by 5 chest thrusts (using 2-finger technique).	
3. Repeat step 2 until the object is expelled (obstruction relieved) or the victim becomes unresponsive.	
Infant Foreign-Body Airway Obstruction — Victim Becomes Unresponsive **The following is for clarification only. It is not to be emphasized or evaluated in the lay rescuer course.**	
4. If a second rescuer is available, send that rescuer to phone 911 (or other emergency response number).	
5. Attempt CPR: each time you open the airway, look for a foreign object in the mouth. If the object is seen, remove it, but *do not perform blind finger sweeps.*	
6. If the infant is unresponsive after about 1 minute of CPR and the rescuer is alone, phone 911 (or other emergency response number), then continue CPR.*	

*If the victim is breathing or resumes normal breathing and no trauma is suspected, place in the recovery position.

Comments _____

_____

_____

Instructor _____

Circle one: Complete   Needs more practice

Heartsaver CPR Course for Infant and Child

Child Foreign-Body Airway Obstruction in Responsive Victim
(and Responsive Victim Who Becomes Unresponsive)
Performance Criteria

American Heart Association®

Fighting Heart Disease and Stroke

Student Name _____ Date _____

Performance Guidelines	Performed
1. Ask "Are you choking?" If the child indicates yes, ask "Can you speak?" If child shakes head "no" or cannot make any sound, tell the child you are going to help. Give abdominal thrusts.	
2. Stand or kneel behind the child and wrap your arms around child. Give abdominal thrusts, avoiding compression on the bottom of the breastbone (xiphoid).	
3. Repeat step 2 until the object is expelled (obstruction relieved) or the victim becomes unresponsive.	
Child Foreign-Body Airway Obstruction — Victim Becomes Unresponsive The following is for clarification only. It is not to be emphasized or evaluated in the lay rescuer course.	
4. If a second rescuer is available, send that rescuer to phone 911 (or other emergency response number).	
5. Attempt CPR (each time you open the airway, open it widely and look for a foreign object in the mouth. If you see an object, remove it, but *do not perform blind finger sweeps*).	
6. If the victim is not responsive after about 1 minute of CPR and the rescuer is alone, phone 911 (or other emergency response number). Continue CPR.*	

*If the victim is breathing or resumes normal breathing and no trauma is suspected, place in the recovery position.

Comments _____
_____
_____

Instructor _____

Circle one: Complete   Needs more practice

Comparison of CPR Rescue Techniques for Adults, Infants, and Children

The most likely cause of cardiac arrest in adults is sudden development of ventricular fibrillation (VF). VF must be treated with defibrillation, and CPR should be performed until defibrillation can be provided. For this reason, *if you are alone,* leave the adult victim to phone 911 and then return to begin CPR. The CPR technique for adults (compression rate of about 100 compressions per minute with a compression-ventilation ratio of 15 to 2) is designed to provide more compressions per minute than are provided for infant or child victims.

In infants less than 6 months old the leading cause of death is SIDS. In infants more than 6 months old and in children the leading cause of death is injury. For this reason the first link in the AHA pediatric Chain of Survival is prevention of injury or arrest. Respiratory arrest precedes cardiac arrest in most infants and children. Delivery of rescue breathing may prevent cardiac arrest. For this reason, *if you are alone* provide about 1 minute of CPR to the unresponsive infant or child and then leave the victim to phone 911 or other emergency response number. The CPR technique for infant and child victims (compression rate of at least 100 compressions per minute for infants and approximately 100 compressions per minute for children, with a compression-ventilation ratio of 5 to 1) is designed to provide more ventilations per minute than are provided to the adult victim.

This difference in the sequence of actions (phone 911 and then begin CPR for adult victims *versus* begin CPR and then phone 911 for infant and child victims) applies only if you are a *lone rescuer.* Whenever other rescuers are present, regardless of the age of the victim, send a second rescuer to phone 911 while you begin CPR.

Critical Concepts

You Find Someone Who Is Unresponsive

Adult Victim	Infant/Child Victim
1. Shout for help.	1. Shout for help.
2. Phone 911.	2. Begin CPR (continue for 1 minute).
3. Begin CPR.	3. Phone 911.

Remember, other rescuers are often nearby. If other rescuers are present, send someone to phone 911 while you begin CPR, regardless of the victim's age.

Summary of Differences Between Adults, Children, and Infants

CPR/Rescue Breathing	Adult and Older Child (more than 8 years old)	Child (1 to 8 years old)	Infant (less than 1 year old)
Establish that victim is unresponsive Activate EMS.	Activate EMS or other emergency response number as soon as victim is found.	Activate EMS or other emergency response number after giving 1 minute of CPR.	Activate EMS or other emergency response number after giving 1 minute of CPR.
Open airway Perform head tilt–chin lift or jaw thrust.	Head tilt–chin lift (If trauma is present, use jaw thrust.)	Head tilt–chin lift (If trauma is present, use jaw thrust.)	Head tilt–chin lift (If trauma is present, use jaw thrust.)
Check for breathing (look, listen, feel) If victim is breathing, place in recovery position. If victim is not breathing normally, give 2 effective slow breaths.			
■ **Initial**	2 effective breaths (2 seconds each)	2 effective breaths (1 to 1½ seconds each)	2 effective breaths (1 to 1½ seconds each)
■ **Subsequent**	10 to 12 breaths per minute (approximate)	20 breaths per minute (approximate)	20 breaths per minute (approximate)
■ **Foreign-body airway obstruction**	Abdominal thrusts	Abdominal thrusts	Back blows or chest thrusts (no abdominal thrusts)
Check for signs of circulation (breathing, coughing, movement, or pulse) If signs of circulation are present, provide airway and breathing support. If no signs of circulation are present, begin chest compressions interposed with breaths.	*Healthcare Providers Only:* ■ Check carotid pulse *Lay Rescuers:* Check for signs of circulation after giving 2 rescue breaths: ■ Normal breathing ■ Coughing ■ Movement If no signs of circulation are present, provide chest compressions.	*Healthcare Providers Only:* ■ Check carotid pulse *Lay Rescuers:* Check for signs of circulation after giving 2 rescue breaths: ■ Normal breathing ■ Coughing ■ Movement If no signs of circulation are present, provide chest compressions.	*Healthcare Providers Only:* ■ Check brachial pulse *Lay Rescuers:* Check for signs of circulation after giving 2 rescue breaths: ■ Normal breathing ■ Coughing ■ Movement If no signs of circulation are present, provide chest compressions.

(Table continued on p. 134)

CPR/Rescue Breathing	Adult and Older Child (more than 8 years old)	Child (1 to 8 years old)	Infant (less than 1 year old)
Compression landmarks	Lower half of sternum (nipple line)	Lower half of sternum	Lower half of sternum (1 finger's width below nipple line)
Compression method	Heel of 1 hand, other hand on top	Heel of 1 hand	2 fingers
Compression depth	1½ to 2 inches	⅓ to ½ the depth of the chest	⅓ to ½ the depth of the chest
Compression rate	Approximately 100 per minute	Approximately 100 per minute	At least 100 per minute
Compression-ventilation ratio	15:2 (1 or 2 rescuers)	5:1 (1 or 2 rescuers)	5:1 (1 or 2 rescuers)

Appendix C

Special Resuscitation Situations

Using the Adult Chain of Survival Sequence for the Infant or Child With Known Heart Disease or Arrhythmias ("Phone First" and Then Begin CPR If You Are Alone)

If a child has known heart disease or is at risk for a sudden arrhythmia that could cause cardiac arrest, the child's doctor or nurse may instruct parents and those who provide care for the child to follow the adult CPR sequence if the child collapses suddenly. The adult Chain of Survival assumes that sudden collapse is caused by a problem with the heart rhythm and is designed to ensure that the EMS system is notified immediately so that a defibrillator arrives at the scene as quickly as possible. If a child with known heart disease collapses, take the following actions:

1. If you determine that the child is unresponsive, shout for help. If another rescuer is present, send that person to phone 911 or other emergency response number.
2. If you are alone, leave the child to phone 911 or other emergency response number. If the child is small and uninjured, bring the child to the phone or the phone to the child so that the dispatcher can guide you through CPR if needed.
3. Begin CPR and provide it as you learned in the Heartsaver CPR Course for Infant and Child.
4. Continue CPR until EMS personnel arrive with equipment to analyze the heart rhythm and treat the arrhythmia if needed.

In reality there is usually more than 1 person at the scene of an emergency. In these cases, if you are the trained rescuer, you should direct someone to phone 911 or other emergency response number while you begin CPR. This allows you to accomplish 2 links of the Chain of Survival at the same time. It is only in the case of a lone (single) rescuer that the sequence of phoning first or beginning CPR first becomes an important issue.

Action Scenarios: Applying Your Knowledge of CPR

This appendix presents study cases to help you learn how to apply the skills of CPR. The following cases review different situations that you may face as a rescuer. Each case illustrates a common emergency that requires a unique action. For each case do the following:

- Cover the answer below the case with a piece of paper and then carefully review the case.
- Jot down the best answer to the case

question. Be prepared to explain your choice in discussions with your instructor.

- Review the correct answer and the discussion of why it is the best answer.
- If the answer and discussion are unclear, review the related section in the manual.
- If you have additional questions, ask your instructor.

CASE 1: A 7-Year-Old Submersion (Near-Drowning) Victim

As you are walking outside a hotel, you hear someone frantically shouting from the area of the hotel swimming pool. A woman has just pulled her child from the swimming pool, and he is not breathing. You run to the pool and see the woman kneeling beside her 7-year-old son. The child is lying at the side of the pool. The woman tells you her son was doing a flip off the diving board and struck his head. What immediate actions should you take?

What is your answer?

_____

_____

Why? _____

_____

_____

Case 1 Answer: Minimum answer is that you must first check to see if the child is responsive. If the child is not responsive, send the woman to phone 911 (or other emergency response number) while you begin CPR.

As you approach the child, be prepared to begin the links in the AHA pediatric Chain of Survival. The child has probably been submerged in the pool, so you can no longer prevent the injury (near-drowning) from occurring (first link).

The next action you must take is to determine whether CPR is necessary. The child may have been "stunned" when striking his head and may respond to simple stimulation. However, the child may be in respiratory or cardiac arrest, so you must be prepared to provide the support the child needs. Your actions will be guided by what you find when you check the child. **Begin by determining whether the child is responsive.** Gently tap the child and call his name. If he does not respond, begin CPR (second link) while you send the mother to phone 911 or other emergency response number (third link).

- Open the airway using a jaw thrust because the child reportedly struck his head when he was diving into the pool. Then look, listen, and feel for breathing.
- If the boy is not breathing normally, give 2 slow rescue breaths, making sure the chest rises with each breath.

- After you give 2 breaths, check for signs of circulation (normal breathing, coughing, or movement in response to the 2 breaths).
- If there are no signs of circulation, begin chest compressions combined with ventilations at a ratio of 5 to 1.

If the child responds very early in this sequence, all these actions will not be necessary.

CASE 2: A 7-Year-Old Submersion (Near-Drowning) Victim (Part 2)

You responded to a woman's shouts for help at a hotel swimming pool. The woman had pulled her 7-year-old son from the pool after he struck his head during a dive. You arrive at the side of the pool and begin to assess the child. You note that he is unresponsive. You immediately begin CPR and send the woman to phone 911. You open the airway and check for breathing. You note that the boy is not breathing and you give 2 slow breaths, ensuring that the chest rises with each breath. You then check for signs of circulation. After the 2 rescue breaths the boy moves his arms and legs but his breathing is inadequate. What action should you take?

What is your answer?

_____

_____

Why? _____

_____

_____

Case 2 Answer: Minimum answer is that you continue rescue breathing at a rate of 1 breath every 3 seconds (about 20 breaths per minute).

Isolated respiratory arrest (the victim stops breathing while maintaining effective circulation) is common to many emergencies, such as near-drowning, head injury, drug overdose or poisoning, and electrocution. Victims who are in respiratory arrest with other signs of circulation (for example, movement) do not require chest compressions. Nevertheless, you should continue to provide rescue breathing and monitor the victim's signs

of circulation until EMS personnel arrive. If the signs of circulation disappear, immediately start chest compressions with rescue breathing at a ratio of 5 compressions to 1 breath. When children and adolescents are involved in drowning emergencies, you should also be concerned about spinal injuries, particularly if the child was diving or struck his head. When attempting to help these victims, be careful to keep the spine in alignment when you remove the victim from the water and use the jaw thrust rather than the head tilt–chin lift to open and maintain the victim's airway.

CASE 3: Emergency at a Fast Food Restaurant

You are eating lunch at a fast food restaurant when you hear an infant cough and gag and then suddenly become silent. The infant's mother jumps from her seat and begins shaking the child and shouts, "Someone help me! She's not breathing and I don't know what to do!" The mother has pulled the infant from the booster seat and is shaking her. The infant is struggling to breathe and her mouth is working, but she is not making a sound. You approach the mother and ask, "Is she choking?" The mother says, "Yes! Please help her! Should you do a Heimlich?" You tell the mother and infant that you are going to try to help. The infant is still making no sounds but appears to be trying to breathe. Her lips are turning blue. What actions should you take?

What is your answer?

_____

_____

Why? _____

_____

_____

Case 3 Answer: Minimum answer: Provide alternating back blows and chest thrusts until the object is expelled or the infant becomes unresponsive.

Tell the mother that you are not performing the Heimlich maneuver but are performing maneuvers recommended by the American Heart Association as appropriate for an infant choking victim. Immediately place the infant face down on your arm, holding the infant's head with your hand and ensuring that the head is lower than the body. To stabilize the infant on your arm, sit in a chair or kneel on the floor. Give up to 5 back blows, and keep watching to see if the obstructing object is expelled. If the object is not expelled after 5 back blows, turn the infant over and give up to 5 chest thrusts. Continue alternating sets of 5 back blows and 5 chest thrusts until the object is expelled or the infant becomes unresponsive.

CASE 4: Infant Choking Victim Becomes Unresponsive

The infant who was choking at the fast food restaurant becomes limp and unresponsive while you are providing back blows and chest thrusts. What actions should you take?

What is your answer?

_____

Why? _____

_____

_____

Case 4 Answer: Minimum answer: You send someone to phone 911 and you begin CPR. Each time you open the airway to attempt ventilation, look for the obstructing object and remove it if you see it.

If the victim becomes unresponsive, send someone to phone 911 while you attempt CPR. Every time you open the airway, open it widely and look for an object. If you see an object in the back of the throat, remove it. If you do not see an object, continue compressions and ventilations (CPR).

- Open the airway widely, look for an object, and remove it if you see it. Look, listen, and feel for breathing.

- If the infant is not breathing normally, give 2 slow breaths. Be sure the chest rises with each breath. If the chest does not rise, reposition the head and airway and reattempt ventilation.
- After delivery of 2 breaths, check for signs of circulation. If there are no signs of circulation (no normal breathing, coughing, or movement in response to your 2 rescue breaths), begin chest compressions.
- Continue cycles of 5 compressions and 1 ventilation. Look in the infant's mouth each time you open the airway to provide ventilations. Remove any foreign object you see.
- Continue CPR until EMS personnel arrive.

CASE 5: Infant Stops Breathing

Friends are visiting from out of town with their 9-month-old infant. The infant has had a virus with high fever, a cough, and a runny nose during the day. The fever has recently been very high. The father is changing the infant and suddenly shouts, "Help! I think she's having a seizure!" You arrive in the room to find the infant jerking in movements that look like a seizure, and then the movements stop. You tap the infant and there is no response. What actions should you take?

What is your answer?

_____

Why? _____

_____

Case 5 Answer: Minimum answer: You should send the father to phone 911 while you begin CPR.

It is likely that this infant had a seizure due to the fever. You have verified that the infant is unresponsive, so you should begin CPR.

- Open the infant's airway, and look, listen, and feel for breathing.
- If the infant is not breathing normally, provide mouth-to-mouth-and-nose (or mouth-to-nose) ventilation and be sure the chest rises with each breath. If the chest does not rise, reopen the airway and reattempt rescue breathing.

- After delivery of 2 breaths, check for signs of circulation. If there is no normal breathing, coughing, or movement in response to the breaths, begin chest compressions at a rate of at least 100 compressions per minute.
- Continue chest compressions and ventilations in a ratio of 5 to 1. Remember to recheck for signs of circulation after 1 minute and every few minutes thereafter until EMS personnel arrive.

It is not uncommon for infants and children to be unresponsive after a seizure. Respiratory arrest may be present. It is very likely that this infant will respond to the 2 rescue breaths and not require chest compressions.

CASE 6: Reducing the Risk of SIDS

A local church begins offering infant care during services. You have volunteered to help in the infant care center. You observe a childcare worker putting an apparently healthy, young infant (2 months old) into a crib for a nap. She places the infant face down on the stomach (prone). What actions should you take?

What is your answer?

_____

_____

Why? _____

_____

_____

Case 6 Answer: Minimum answer: You should tell the childcare worker that healthy infants should be placed on their back or side to sleep because this reduces the risk of sudden infant death syndrome.

SIDS is the death of a young infant, usually during the first 6 months of life, that is unexplained by the infant's medical history or other causes even when an autopsy is performed. The risk of SIDS is increased in infants who sleep in the prone position (on their stomach). For this reason all healthy infants should be placed on their back or side to sleep. If they are placed on their side, they should be propped to prevent them from rolling onto their stomach. This recommendation is easy to remember: "Place your infant **back** to sleep."

CASE 7: Prevention of Child Injuries and Cardiac Arrest

You are transporting a group of 7-year-old children to a school event. Three of the children are at least 58 inches tall, and they climb into the back seat of the van and put on lap and shoulder belts. The shoulder belts cross from their shoulders, across the breastbone to the pelvis, and the lap belts fit snugly across their hips. A fourth child climbs into the front seat and puts on the lap and shoulder belt; the shoulder belt crosses the child's neck no matter how much you adjust the belt on its frame. What actions should you take?

What is your answer?

_____

Why? _____

_____

Case 7 Answer: Minimum answer: Tell the child that he or she must sit in the back seat and must use a belt-positioning booster seat (assuming you have one) to ensure that he or she is properly restrained.

Motor vehicle crashes are the leading cause of fatal injury in children. Children must be appropriately restrained for their age. Lap and shoulder belts are appropriate for children only if they are taller than 4 ft, 9 inches (58 inches; 148 cm) and weigh 80 pounds (36 kg) and can sit in the seat with their legs comfortably bent over the edge of the seat. In addition, the lap belt should cross from the shoulder, across the breastbone to the pelvis. If the shoulder harness crosses the child's neck, the belt should be adjusted. If the belt cannot be adjusted, the child must be placed in a belt-positioning booster seat. In addition, if the car has a passenger-side airbag, children 12 years old or younger should sit in the back seat.

Appendix E

Glossary of Terms

Artery — A blood vessel that carries blood away from the heart to the various parts of the body.

Automated External Defibrillator (AED) — A computerized medical device that identifies irregular ("shockable") heart rhythms, specifically ventricular tachycardia and ventricular fibrillation. If a shockable rhythm is detected, the AED charges to an appropriate shock dose and advises the operator to deliver an electric shock to a victim of cardiac arrest in an attempt to allow a normal heart rhythm to resume. An AED can be operated by lay rescuers and used for adults and children older than 8 years of age in cardiac arrest (no response, no normal breathing, no signs of circulation). The AED assesses the victim's cardiac rhythm to determine whether a rhythm that will respond to shocks is present. If such a rhythm is detected, the AED "advises" the operator to press the SHOCK button. See **Defibrillator**.

Barrier Devices — Plastic or silicon devices that allow a rescuer to provide rescue breathing without directly touching the victim's mouth or nose. The devices are placed over the victim's mouth and nose. There are 2 types: *face shields*, which are flexible and mold closely to the face, and *face masks*, which are rigid and increase the distance between the victim and rescuer.

Blood Pressure — The force of pressure exerted by the heart in pumping blood; the pressure of blood in the arteries.

Cardiac Arrest — A condition in which the heart suddenly stops pumping blood. Sudden cardiac arrest in adults is most often caused by an abnormal heart rhythm (usually ventricular fibrillation).

The victim in cardiac arrest demonstrates no response to stimuli, no normal breathing, and no signs of circulation (no normal breathing, coughing, or movement in response to 2 rescue breaths).

Cardiopulmonary Resuscitation (CPR) — A series of steps that include opening the airway, assessing breathing, providing rescue breathing, assessing signs of circulation, and providing chest compressions. These actions keep oxygen-rich blood flowing to the brain until defibrillation attempts and advanced life support can be provided.

Cardiovascular — Pertaining to the heart and blood vessels, including the major blood vessels that supply blood to the brain.

Circulatory System — The heart and blood vessels (arteries, veins, and capillaries).

Defibrillation — Successful treatment of ventricular fibrillation using electric shocks delivered by a defibrillator.

Defibrillator — A medical device that delivers electric shocks (electric current) to the heart to treat ventricular fibrillation. The current is delivered through either adhesive electrode pads attached to the chest or through handheld metal paddles. Defibrillators can be either automated or manual. Manual defibrillators are operated by healthcare providers, but automated external defibrillators (AEDs) can be operated by lay rescuers in communities with programs of public access defibrillation or by healthcare providers. See **Automated External Defibrillator**.

Endotracheal Tube or Tracheal Tube — A plastic tube inserted from the mouth into the windpipe of a victim who is not breathing effectively (may be called a "breathing tube"). Advanced healthcare personnel (doctors, nurses, and paramedics) may insert these tubes.

Heart Attack — A nonspecific term usually referring to complete blockage of a diseased coronary artery by a blood clot that results in injury to and often death of the heart muscle supplied by that artery. *Myocardial infarction* is a more specific term for what is usually meant by *heart attack.*

Myocardium — Heart muscle.

Public Access Defibrillation (PAD) — A public health initiative developed by the American Heart Association. PAD encourages the development of programs that provide automated external defibrillators (AEDs) throughout the community and rescuers trained to use them. PAD programs require physician supervision and contact with the local emergency medical services (EMS) system. In communities with a PAD program, AEDs can be used by a large number of rescuers, including firefighters, police officers, security guards, and even family members of high-risk patients. Quick, accurate use of an AED can substantially shorten the time to defibrillation and improve the chance of survival of victims of out-of-hospital cardiac arrest.

Pulmonary — Pertaining to the lungs.

Respiratory Arrest — A condition in which a victim is not breathing at all or is breathing so slowly, shallowly, or irregularly that adequate oxygenation of the blood cannot occur. To distinguish it from *cardiac arrest,* this term is reserved for victims who are not breathing effectively but who still have signs of circulation.

Sudden Infant Death Syndrome (SIDS) — The sudden death of an infant, typically between the ages of 1 month and 1 year, that is not explained by the infant's medical history or other causes even when an autopsy (postmortem examination) is performed. SIDS probably includes a variety of conditions that result in death during sleep. Many factors are associated with an increased risk of SIDS, including a prone sleeping position (on the stomach).

Vascular — Pertaining to the blood vessels.

Vein — Any one of a series of vessels of the cardiovascular system that carry blood from various parts of the body back to the heart.

Ventricular Fibrillation (VF) — A chaotic, uncoordinated quivering of the cardiac muscle that prevents effective contraction of the heart. VF causes cardiac arrest; biological death follows within minutes if VF is not treated. Defibrillation is the treatment needed for VF. A defibrillator is used to deliver a strong electric shock to the heart. When this shock is successful, the heart is "stunned," and a normal rhythm resumes (defibrillation has occurred).

Appendix F

Frequently Asked Questions About CPR

1. *Can rescuers catch AIDS, hepatitis, or other diseases during CPR?*

It is extremely unlikely that a rescuer will become infected with human immunodeficiency virus (HIV), the virus that causes AIDS, or any of the hepatitis viruses as a result of performing mouth-to-mouth breathing or touching the victim. CPR (including mouth-to-mouth breathing) has been performed for more than 35 years, and there has never been a documented case of transmission of HIV or any hepatitis virus from a victim to a rescuer. You can use a face mask or a face shield as a barrier device, but such a device is not necessary to perform CPR. The face shield prevents contact with the victim's mouth and face. The mask contains a 1-way valve to help block transmission of viruses and bacteria.

It is important for rescuers to know that most (70% to 80%) respiratory and cardiac arrests in infants and children occur in and around the home, where the rescuer usually knows the victim and knows about the victim's health conditions. A primary reason to learn CPR is for the benefit of your family and friends. Barrier devices should be available for all rescuers who provide CPR in the workplace.

2. *What are some possible hazards of CPR?*

CPR can cause injuries, but such injuries have been reported much more frequently in adult victims than in infant and child victims. Follow performance guidelines at all times to reduce the risk of potential complications of CPR. Frequent practice with a manikin helps improve future performance. Possible problems in performing CPR that may contribute to complications include the following:

- Incorrect positioning of the hands for chest compressions may lead to rib fractures, fractures of the end of the breastbone (xiphoid), and bruising or bleeding of the liver, lung, or spleen.
- Bouncing chest compressions may cause the rescuer's hands to move off the center of the sternum (breastbone) so that other structures (ribs, lung, liver) are compressed and possibly injured.
- Compressing the chest too deeply may cause internal injury.
- Not compressing the sternum deeply enough may provide insufficient blood flow to the brain and other vital organs.
- Providing a volume of breath that is too great, breathing too rapidly, or not opening the airway completely may cause you to blow large amounts of air into the stomach and cause the stomach to fill with air (gastric inflation). Gastric inflation increases the chances that the victim will vomit and may decrease the effectiveness of ventilations.

3. *How do I open the airway of a victim who may have a neck injury, such as a victim of a car crash?*

Use a jaw thrust to open the airway of a victim suspected of having a neck injury.

4. *What should I do if the victim vomits?*

If the victim vomits, turn the victim's head and body to the side so that the victim will not choke on the vomited material. If you suspect a head or neck injury, turn the head, neck, and entire body to the side as a unit ("log roll") without flexing or turning the neck. Then clear the airway by sweeping the mouth. A cloth (for example, a corner of clothing or handkerchief) wrapped around your fingers can be used to sweep the mouth. Then reposition the victim and continue CPR. If you suspect an injury to the head or neck, you *must* turn the head, neck, and body as one unit.

5. *How will I know if signs of circulation and breathing return?*

The return of signs of circulation, with or without breathing, may be dramatic or subtle. The victim may take a big gasp of air, begin moving, cough, or even start to become responsive. If normal breathing returns, keep the airway open and regularly check for signs of circulation and breathing. Place the victim in a recovery position to maintain an open airway. If an infant or child victim is not breathing normally (for example, occasional attempts at gasping are made), perform rescue breathing at a rate of about 20 breaths per minute (about once every 3 seconds).

6. *What should I do if an infant or a child with a tracheostomy needs CPR?*

Children who have a tracheostomy have a permanent opening (stoma) that connects the airway or windpipe (trachea) directly to the skin of the neck. The opening is at the base of the front of the neck. In most children with a tracheostomy a tube is placed in the tracheostomy to keep the airway open. To tell whether the victim's breathing has returned, place your ear over the opening in the neck. If rescue breathing is required, perform mouth-to-tracheostomy-tube rescue breathing. If you cannot get air to enter the tube, the tube itself may be blocked, and it may be necessary to remove the tube and provide mouth-to-stoma ventilation. For more information, contact the International Association of Laryngectomees, ℅ American Cancer Society, 1599 Clifton Rd NE, Atlanta, GA 30329.

7. *If a victim is lying on a bed, should I move him to the floor so that a hard surface is under his back?*

Victims who need CPR should be moved to a firm level surface if at all possible, so you should move the victim to the floor. Make sure that the victim's head and neck are well supported. In general, you should be able to move an infant or child to the floor or to a sturdy table (for example, a changing table). However, if you are alone and cannot move the victim, leave the victim on the bed and try to find something flat and firm (such as an ironing board or other board) to slide under the victim's back to provide a firm surface. If you cannot immediately locate something to place under the victim and you absolutely cannot move the victim, begin CPR with the victim on the bed (do not delay). Try to compress the chest with enough force that the breastbone moves inward about one third to one half the depth of the chest.

8. *What should I do to prevent air from filling the stomach (gastric inflation)?*

Inflation of the stomach (air getting into the stomach) is most likely to occur if you blow too hard during rescue breathing or if the airway is partially obstructed. Control the force and speed of rescue breaths. Breathe slowly into the victim, taking 1 to 1½ seconds to deliver each breath, and blow only enough air to make the victim's chest rise slightly.

9. *How will I know when to perform abdominal thrusts for a child victim who is choking?*

If the victim can cough forcefully and make sounds, the victim is moving air and does not have complete airway obstruction, so abdominal thrusts are unnecessary. You may hear wheezing between coughs. As long as good air exchange continues, encourage the victim to keep coughing and breathing. At this point do not interfere with the victim's attempts to expel the foreign object. With severe or complete airway obstruction, the child will be unable to speak, breathe, or cough forcefully. The victim also may clutch her neck (universal sign of choking). If the victim cannot speak or make a sound, try to relieve the obstruction with abdominal thrusts (the Heimlich maneuver).

10. *How often should I review or renew my skills in CPR?*

The AHA Emergency Cardiovascular Care Committee recommends retraining at least every 2 years to renew CPR skills. The committee encourages you to practice your CPR skills frequently within this time period, however.

Appendix G
Self-Test Questions

Please take the following self-test. If you are unsure of an answer, review the material on the pages listed below the item.

1. **Which infant sleeping position is associated with the lowest risk of sudden infant death syndrome (SIDS)?**

   a. prone position
   b. lying on a fluffy comforter or lamb's wool
   c. lying on the back
   d. lying on the stomach

   Answer is **c**; see pages 83-84.

2. **You discover your 3-year-old nephew lying limp on the bathroom floor. An empty pill bottle is beside him. You gently shake him and shout, "Are you OK?" He does not respond. You shout for help but no one comes. What do you do next?**

   a. give 2 rescue breaths
   b. perform a head tilt–chin lift and look, listen, and feel for breathing
   c. leave him to phone 911
   d. check for signs of circulation

   Answer is **b**; see pages 102-103.

3. **You have opened your nephew's airway, confirmed that he is not breathing, and given 2 slow rescue breaths (1 to 1½ seconds per breath). What do you do next?**

   a. get an AED
   b. perform a head tilt–chin lift and look, listen, and feel for breathing
   c. perform chest compressions
   d. check for signs of circulation

   Answer is **d**; see page 105.

4. **You observe signs of circulation (your 3-year-old nephew coughs and breathes occasionally), but he is breathing very slowly, shallowly, and irregularly. What do you do next?**

   a. perform rescue breathing with a compression ("pumping") to breathing ("blowing") ratio of 15:2
   b. perform rescue breathing with a compression ("pumping") to breathing ("blowing") ratio of 5:1
   c. perform rescue breathing at a rate of 1 breath every 3 seconds
   d. place him in the recovery position to maintain an open airway

   Answer is **c**; see pages 103-104.

5. **You are alone and you have performed rescue breathing for your nephew for about 1 minute. What do you do next?**

   a. place him in the recovery position
   b. phone 911 or other emergency response number
   c. check for signs of circulation
   d. give 2 rescue breaths

   Answer is **b**; see page 102.

6. **You return to your nephew and continue rescue breathing. After several minutes of rescue breathing, he coughs and then begins to breathe regularly. What do you do next?**

   a. perform a head tilt–chin lift and look, listen, and feel for breathing
   b. place him in the recovery position and continue to monitor his breathing
   c. begin chest compressions and check for signs of circulation every few minutes
   d. give 2 rescue breaths

   Answer is **b**; see page 105.

7. **You are at the food court in a shopping mall. A 10-month-old who has been eating his brother's french fries suddenly begins to cough repeatedly and appears to be in distress. What do you do next?**

   a. phone 911 or other emergency response number
   b. perform a head tilt–chin lift and look, listen, and feel for breathing
   c. perform 5 back blows and 5 chest thrusts until the object is expelled or the infant becomes unresponsive
   d. monitor for signs of complete airway obstruction and be prepared to act if they develop

   Answer is **d**; see page 109.

8. **The infant's 7-year-old brother is also eating french fries. He begins to cough forcefully and has very noisy breath sounds. Suddenly he becomes silent even though he is still trying to breathe. He clutches his throat, does not speak, and looks alarmed. What should you do next?**

   a. phone 911 or other emergency response number
   b. ask, "Are you choking?"
   c. perform abdominal thrusts
   d. do not interfere but monitor the situation

   Answer is **b**; see page 110.

9. **You see a 5-year-old on the school playground fall head first from the top of a tall slide, striking her head on the ground. You run to her side and find she is unresponsive. You send one of the teachers to phone 911. What do you do next?**

   a. open the airway with a jaw thrust and look, listen, and feel for breathing
   b. do nothing unless you have a barrier device with you
   c. open the airway with a head tilt–chin lift and look, listen, and feel for breathing
   d. place her in the recovery position

   Answer is **a**; see pages 102-103.